Keto Diet

The Step by Step Keto Cookbook

To Gain Ketosis

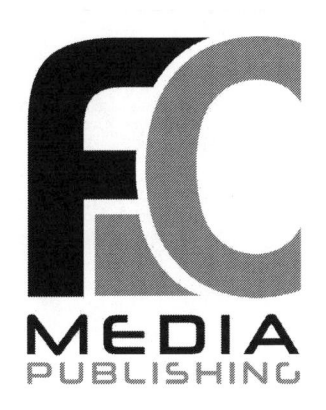

Jamie Ken Moore

© Copyright 2018 by Jamie Ken Moore - All rights reserved.

This document is geared towards providing exact and reliable information in regards to the topic and issue covered. The publication is sold with the idea that the publisher is not required to render accounting, officially permitted, or otherwise, qualified services. If advice is necessary, legal or professional, a practiced individual in the profession should be ordered.

From a Declaration of Principles which was accepted and approved by a Committee of the American Bar Association and a Committee of Publishers and Associations.

In no way is it legal to reproduce, duplicate, or transmit any part of this document in either electronic means or in printed format. Recording of this publication is strictly prohibited and any storage of this document is not allowed unless with written permission from the publisher. All rights reserved.

The information provided herein is stated to be truthful and consistent, in that any liability, in terms of inattention or otherwise, by any usage or abuse of any policies, processes, or directions contained within is the solitary and utter responsibility of the recipient reader. Under no circumstances will any legal responsibility or blame be held against the publisher for any reparation, damages, or monetary loss due to the information herein, either directly or indirectly.

Respective authors own all copyrights not held by the publisher.

The information herein is offered for informational purposes solely, and is universal as so. The presentation of the information is without contract or any type of guarantee assurance.

The trademarks that are used are without any consent, and the publication of the trademark is without permission or backing by the trademark owner. All trademarks and brands within this book are for clarifying purposes only and are owned by the owners themselves, not affiliated with this document.

Table of Contents

INTRODUCTION 1

CHAPTER 1 THE SECRETS OF THE KETOGENIC DIET PLAYBOOK 3

CHAPTER 2 THE YES AND NO OF KETO FOODS 14

CHAPTER 3 A KETO HELPER: THE 28 DAY MEAL PLAN 23

CHAPTER 4 STEP BY STEP: HIGH FAT LOW CARB KETO RECIPES 28

Breakfast 32

Lunch 52

Dinner 76

Fat Bombs, Snacks And Desserts 94

CONCLUSION: TIME TO TAKE ACTION AND GET KETOGENIC 117

ABOUT THE AUTHOR. 118

APPENDIX A: THE GROCERY LISTS 119

APPENDIX B: CONVERSION CHARTS 127

APPENDIX C: RECIPE INDEX 128

This page has been intentionally left blank

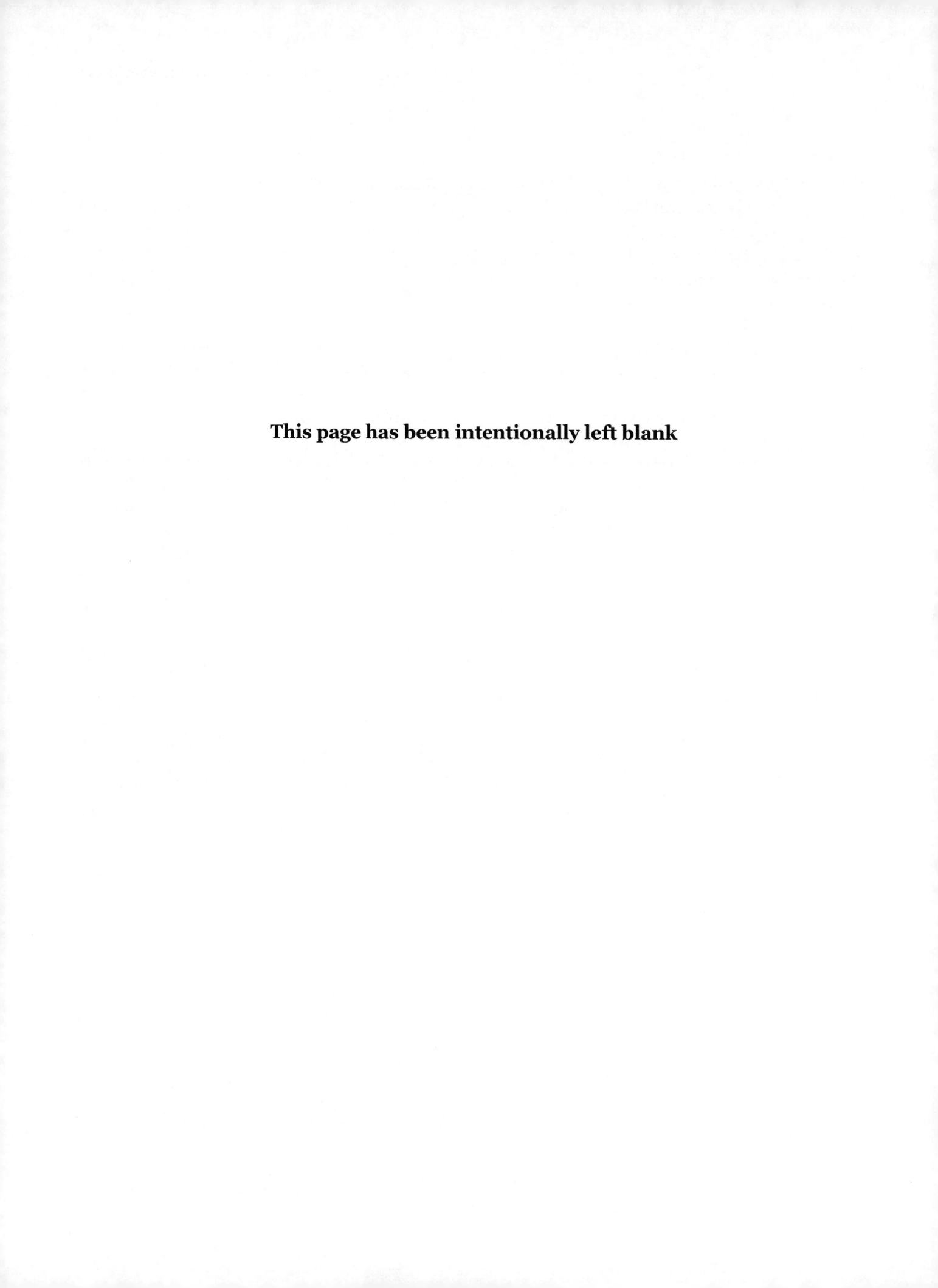

Introduction

Have you been wanting to get to work on that physique but felt that you had to lose some weight first? Or could it be that the term "weight loss" has been hanging around in the back of your mind, just that you never really got down to working on it? Restrictive and strange diets, fanciful expensive machines, and the ultimate fat-burning, no-workout magic weight loss pill. These would be the many purported solutions that one would find whenever you seek an answer in the dazzling, multi-billion dollar weight loss industry.

The truth is, by coming to this book, you already have an inkling of what is truly needed to effect safe and lasting weight loss. It is a natural fact that only through watching what we eat, will we have the most impact on our weight. This is where the ketogenic diet really shines and lets you enjoy automatic, effortless fat burning without all the usual calorie constraints of other diets.

Weight loss is an almost certain result you will enjoy once you start the ketogenic diet, but this is not the only benefit that you will enjoy. Think of all those activities you have always wanted to pursue, but shelved because you simply had no energy left after your usual day's work. Well, time to dust off those hobbies and the things you enjoy doing, because on the ketogenic diet, you will have more energy for your daily work and play! The accompanying mental clarity and sharpness of thought are also positive effects which you will have as a direct result of the diet. A better health report card, by way of optimized cholesterol readings, normalized blood sugar and a corresponding lowered risk of cardiovascular diseases are also just some of the beneficial health effects experienced by most on the diet.

This book's aim is primarily to give you the tools with which to let the ketogenic diet run more smoothly and seamlessly in your daily life. Something that many learn is that a diet is almost only as good as the number of recipes it has in its repertoire. The benefits of a particular diet may be numerous, but if you are forced to have the same stuff every breakfast, lunch and dinner, even the most avid supporter of the lot would probably have problems sustaining the diet. This is where I am most happy to say that the ketogenic diet has quite some leeway for the concoction of various different recipes, and it is the purpose of this book to bring you some of the more delicious and easy-to-prepare meals for your gastronomic pleasure!

For the beginners as well as the adepts of the ketogenic diet, the recipes contained within are created specifically to be appealing to your palate while not requiring you to literally spend the whole day in the kitchen! Concise and to the point, the recipes break down meal preparation requirements in a simple step by step format, easy for anyone to understand. An additional 28-day meal plan is also structured to serve both as guidance as well as inspiration for the new and old adherents to the ketogenic diet. Grocery lists top it all off to give you the timely reminder on what to get on your next food shopping trip.

The very fact that you are here with this book, is sufficient proof that you are at least curious to know how the ketogenic diet can help you. Even better, maybe you are already quite well-versed with its benefits and are seeking diverse, rich, and savory recipes for a more delectable ketogenic journey.

Regardless of which is which, this keto diet cookbook will be well placed to provide you with actionable culinary ideas with which to spice up your daily meals.

I really hope that the value and ideas you find in this book will serve you well, and may you have a fruitful ketogenic journey!

Chapter 1
The Secrets Of The Ketogenic Diet Playbook

What You Need To Know About The Ketogenic Diet

The ketogenic diet, otherwise known as the keto diet, is not a new-fangled fad diet based on shaky nutritional science. It has been around since the olden times, with ancient Greeks utilizing the diet as part of a holistic treatment for epilepsy. In fact, over here in the States, it was an acknowledged means of treatment for childhood epileptic seizures throughout the 1920s. Unfortunately, this natural way of therapy had to give way to the modern advances of pharmaceutical science with its penchant for immediate effects.

Happily, the ketogenic diet has found its way back into the mainstream yet again and probably for very good reasons! You see, the basis of the diet is to essentially trigger your body's own fat burning mechanisms in order to fuel what the body requires for energy throughout the day. This means that the fat that you eat, as well as the stored fat in your body, have all become fuel stores your body can tap on! Little wonder that this diet really helps you with weight loss, even for those stubborn, hard to lose fatty areas. That could be one of the reasons why you picked this book and looked into embarking on the ketogenic journey, or you may have heard stuff from your social circle about how the keto diet actually normalizes blood sugar levels as well as optimizes your cholesterol readings and you are intrigued. How about stories of type 2 diabetes being reversed just through following this diet alone, as well as tales of certain cancers being halted or the tumors shrinking due to the positive effects of the keto diet? We must also not forget the accompanying risk reduction of cardiovascular disease as a result of the diet!

All of the benefits mentioned above stem largely from a single important process in the ketogenic diet. Ketosis is the name of the game.

Ketosis Know-How

Ketosis is a state where the body produces molecules called ketones which are created by the liver. Designed to give energy to the cells and organs, it can replace glucose as an alternate fuel source. In our traditional carbohydrate-rich diet, we get most of our energy from glucose, which is converted from the carbs that we eat during meals. Glucose is a quick source of energy, where insulin is required as a sort of messenger that tells the cells to open up and allow glucose to flow in such that it can be used as fuel for the mitochondria, otherwise known as the energy factories in our cells.

The more carbs we ingest, the more glucose will be present in our blood, which then means the pancreas needs to produce more insulin in order to facilitate energy production from the available blood sugar. In a body where the metabolic function is still normal, the insulin produced from the pancreas is readily accepted by the cells, which then leads to an efficient usage of blood sugar as energy. The problem is that our cells can actually become insulin desensitized, leading to a situation where the pancreas is forced to pump more and more insulin into the body just to clear and normalize the blood sugar levels.

Insulin de-sensitivity or insulin resistance is created mainly due to the continual elevated presence of glucose in the blood, usually caused by the ingestion of carb-rich foods. Think of your body's cells as a bouncer at a club, where entry to the club requires that you pay a fee. You play the role of glucose here, and the fee required to enter the club is insulin. If your frequency to the club is in line with the norm, the bouncer does not detect anything unusual and so does not raise the fee required for entry. However, if you show up just about every night clamoring to be let in, the bouncer knows your desperate need and correspondingly jacks up the insulin fee in order to let the glucose in. Gradually, the entry fee becomes higher and higher until such a point where the source of insulin, which in this case is the pancreas, no longer produces any. This is where the situation will be diagnosed as type 2 diabetes, and the usual solution would entail being on a lifetime of meds or insulin shots.

The crux of the matter here lies in the presence of glucose in the body system. Every time we take in a carb-rich meal, which isn't difficult in this day and age of fast food and sugary treats, our blood sugar levels get elevated and insulin is activated for the conversion into energy as well as storage of the unused excess into fat cells. This is where the usual furor arises, with condemnations coming in for both glucose and insulin as being the root of many diseases and dreaded weight gain. I would like to take this opportunity to state that insulin and glucose are most definitely not the root of all evil, as some books have made them out to be. It would be far more accurate to point to our current diet as being the leading cause of obesity and metabolic diseases plaguing the better part of the developed world.

Cue the ketogenic diet, which is where we can see the change for the better. The keto diet is a fat-based diet, with an emphasis on being deliberately low carb. This approach is designed so that we reduce our intake of sugary and starchy foods which are so conveniently available. Just a fun fact: sugar was actually used as a preservative in the olden days, and it is no coincidence that much of the processed foods we see today contain high amounts of sugar just because it allows for a lengthened shelf life. Foods high in sugar have also been shown to trigger the hedonic hunger response in the brain, essentially causing you to eat for the sake of pleasure rather than real hunger. Studies have shown that sugary treats are linked to the areas of the brain which are also responsible for gambling and drug addiction. Now you know why you can't seem to stop popping those candied sweets into your mouth!

So we cut down on the carbs, and this is where fats come in to replace the energy needed to sustain the body. On the standard ketogenic diet, you will be looking to take in 75% of your daily calories as fats, about 20% of it as proteins and the remaining 5% in the form of carbs. We do this because, as you remember, we want fats to become our principal source of fuel. Only with the combination of cutting down carbs and increasing our fat intake will we trigger the body to initiate ketosis. Its either we do it through the diet which allows long term and sustainable usage, or we actually starve ourselves into ketosis. Yep, you heard me right, ketosis is the body's natural function that builds a buffer against those lean times when food is scarce.

Keto Diet A Starvation Diet?

This has been also bandied around a lot in recent times, with some trying to cast a negative light on the keto diet by dint of associating it with starvation. To make things clear, the process of ketosis is triggered when our bodies sense we do not have sufficient glucose in the system. It then turns to our fat stores to convert them into ketones through the liver in order to maintain continued energy supply for our cells and organs. It does not mean that on the keto diet, you are actually starving yourself! I get a little worked up every time somebody says that. How can a person taking in 1,800 to 2,000 calories on a daily basis, which is what you will get on the meal plan, be effectively starving?

To be fair, ketosis came in really handy during the hunter-gatherer times of our human history. This was a period where agriculture wasn't that wide spread, and the food you ate depended on what you hunted or found. This created a situation where there might be no food for days at a time, so when glucose found its way into the system, our bodies dispatched insulin to ferry it into our organs as well as hoard the unused glucose into fat cells for future use.

During the lean times when there really was no food to be had, the body then entered the state of ketosis by utilizing the stored fats to supply energy. During this state, our hunger hormones like ghrelin, get their production reduced, and the hormones which control satiety, like leptin, see their levels elevated. All this is because our bodies are trying to make the best of things and allow us to be as comfortable as possible when it detects that food sources are scarce.

Now, fast forward to modern times, when food is literally just one or two blocks, or maybe just a car's drive away, and we probably won't face food shortages like our Paleolithic ancestors. Our bodies, though, still contain the processes and mechanisms which enabled them to survive. That is the key reason why, on the keto diet, we cut carbs and increase our daily fat intake. When we do that, the state of ketosis is induced, and we get to enjoy all the metabolic benefits which the diet confers. The fat that we eat also goes into replenishing the fat stores in the body, which is why I have to say again, you do not starve while on the ketogenic diet!

Once this point is made, some folks then zone in on the multimillion-dollar question. If eating fats get stored as fat, why do we almost always lose weight when on the keto diet?

How Keto Brings Weight Loss

One of the first things that we always lose when we embark on the ketogenic diet is most definitely water weight. The body stores glucose as adipose fats, but there is a small supply of glucose that is stored as glycogen, which consists of mostly water. Glycogen is meant to supply quick bursting energy, the sort that we need when we are sprinting or lifting weights. As we cut carbs, the body turns to glycogen as the first pool of energy supply, which is why water weight will be lost in the initial stages. This initial burst of lost weight can be a morale booster for many, and it is a good portent for what is to come for folks who stick to the keto diet. On a side note, water weight is easily lost, and gained. This means that for folks who see some results on the keto diet initially and then decide to get off the bandwagon for some reason, the chances are their weight would balloon back up once carbs becomes the daily caloric mainstay.

For the rest who stick with the ketogenic diet, what happens next will be the body's fat burning mechanism which is responsible for the astounding weight loss results seen by many. The basic premise is still the same, in that adipose fats are now activated as sources of energy by the body's organs and cells, leading to a natural state of fat loss and hence accompanying weight reduction.

Fat burning is not the only reason why weight loss is seen on the keto diet. Hunger suppression and improve satiety after meals are also reasons why folks are able to lose weight better whilst on the diet. The adage of eating less and moving more has always been one of the long standing tenets in weight loss. The whole idea is to create a calorie deficit such that the body is required to rely on its stored supplies of energy to make up for the required expenditure. On paper, that sounds easy and simple, but for anyone who has been through situations where you have had to consciously curb your eating on a hungry stomach, it could be as difficult as scaling Mount Everest!

With the ketogenic diet, you know that you will have natural hunger suppression, due to the adjustment of the hormones which control feelings of hunger and fullness. Besides that, the food that we typically consume whilst on the diet also helps out with the weight loss. Fats and protein are known to be more satiating and fulfilling than sugary carbs. When we switch to a high fat diet while cutting down on the carbs, we achieve two things pretty much at the same time. Easing back on carbs, especially the sugary stuff, reduces the impulse to eat just because you feel like it, not because you are truly hungry. Jacking up the fat intake also creates the satiety effect much quicker and lets you feel full. This is part of the reason why many keto dieters say that they can go on two and a half or even two meals a day without feeling the slightest pinch of hunger.

On our keto meal plan, we account for a daily caloric intake that ranges from 1,800 to 2,000 calories, so we do not really utilize calorie restriction in order to reduce weight. The reality is that, when you are experiencing fullness and satisfaction from your meals, those tiny and innocent looking snacks that occupy the time in between meals will not feature much in your life! Think about it: donuts, chips, and cakes, which are the typical go-to snacks, get cut out, simply because you are less likely to give in to hedonistic hunger caused primarily by those same sugary treats! That goes a really long way in cutting excess calories which would otherwise have been converted to adipose fat tissue.

To sum it up, the ketogenic diet allows for meals without the typical calorie restriction of other weight loss diets. It also gives a helping hand in creating hunger suppression effects so that you do not have to contend with those dastardly hunger pangs! There is also the absence of carb cravings, which can potentially derail any diet. This lets us enjoy natural weight loss with as little disruption to our daily lives as possible. No calorie counters need to be deployed, no need for a troublesome six to eight meals a day, and definitely no weird or funny exercise routines required. When you couple that with the fulfilling keto high fat meals, you reach a situation where hunger might get to become a stranger indeed.

Getting to relearn what true hunger is like also comes as another positive spin off. On a carb-rich diet, we get instances of hunger because our blood sugar levels tend to fluctuate wildly as our cells become gradually insulin desensitized. Sugar also increases the tendency to eat on impulse, which can really derail any diet! When we cut down on carbs and ramp up on the fats, we would really have to sit up and take notice when we feel any hunger pangs, because those would be proper signals that your body needs refueling.

High Fat Or No Fat

This topic is sure to come up when we are talking about the ketogenic diet. Fat has always been vilified as one of the main causes of cardiovascular disease. This was in no small part due to the Seven

Countries Study done by Ancel Keys where he corroborated research findings from seven different countries that ultimately caused him to link consumption of fat with increased risk of cardiovascular ailments. It was a classic case of just focusing on research numbers which supported his hypothesis, and disregarding the other portions which might have contradicted his theory.

This study led to a literal worldwide clamp down on fat consumption and low fat diets, if you remember those, became all the rage. Thankfully, current research has at least debunked some of the link between fats and heart problems. What most modern scientists and nutritionists can agree on is that there are some fats which are not harmful to the body. In fact, fats are termed as an essential macronutrient, precisely because our bodies need them to function. Let us now take a look at the fats which are deemed beneficial to the human system, because they will be important components of the ketogenic diet!

Monounsaturated fats, of which I shall not bore you with the stuffy chemical definition, are usually present in liquid form at room temperature in their purest state but will tend to solidify when you place them in chilly confines. You would be hard pressed to find anyone who gives a negative review on this particular fat these days, because it has been classified as a heart healthy fat. A little bit of irony is at play here, since it wasn't too long ago that all fats were labelled as one of the main causes of heart disease, and right now, we have the monounsaturated type actually responsible for lowering the risks of cardiac problems!

Most of the monounsaturated fats that we consume come in the form of avocados as well as olive oil. It is also present in almonds, cashew nuts, as well as eggs. Another source of monounsaturated fat, which would probably become one of our intuitive choices of food, would be dark chocolate. Remember, we are talking about chocolate where the cocoa content is at least 80% - the higher the better. Dark chocolate may take some getting used to, especially for folks with a sweet tooth who like milk chocolate. The difference in the impact on health, however, makes it all worthwhile to embrace the switch. Without the excess sugars present, and with a corresponding increase in the beneficial cocoa content, dark chocolate helps with lowering bad LDL cholesterol as well as improving the cardiac risk profile of the consumer. Besides the beneficial monounsaturated fats, dark chocolate also contains a rich level of helpful antioxidants which work to curb chronic inflammatory diseases as well as improve cognitive function.

Another fat which has received some positive scientific literature would be the polyunsaturated variety. Like its monounsaturated sibling, it is normally found in liquid form at room temperature, while refrigeration would generally solidify these fats. Polyunsaturated fats are much more susceptible to oxidation from heat and light, and this is where the crux of the problem lies. Oils from soybean and corn, as well as the sunflower, are rich sources of omega-6 polyunsaturated fatty acids, and these fats are supposed to lower your LDL cholesterol. However, it is common to have both heat and light in copious quantities when we examine most oil extraction methods. The same would also hold true for fish oils which are rich in omega-3, the other famous polyunsaturated fatty acid. Problems in processing, which entail too much heat and light, inevitably oxidizes the erstwhile healthy fats.

When oxidized, the polyunsaturated fat becomes a totally different animal. Oxidized fats are known as trans fats, or franken fats. They bring absolutely no health benefits to the body but dramatically increase cardiovascular risk incidence as well as boosting carcinogenic growth within the body. Free radical levels are also elevated when we consume trans fats. If there were a substance on earth that I would not recommend, this would probably top the list. To make things worse, trans fats only occur in infinitesimal quantities naturally, which means we probably wouldn't suffer from its effects if we just left things to nature. Unfortunately, most of the trans fats wrecking their way into our body systems are of human construct, by way of oil extraction and processing. Most of the fried and processed foods available in the market are also derivatives of vegetable oil, due to its cheap and ready availability. We would do ourselves a big favor if we were to really steer clear of these vegetable oils. Instead, there are certain oils and substances which are more suitable for high heat cooking and we shall definitely touch on those later.

For now though, our best bet for getting quality, unadulterated omega-6 and omega-3 polyunsaturated fatty acids would probably be through eating unprocessed pine nuts and pistachios. Fatty fish like trout and salmon would be great sources of omega-3, taken raw in the Japanese sashimi style or lightly grilled in Mediterranean flavors would also be good. For the folks who are thinking about getting omega-3 supplements like fish oil, it would be best if you could go for producers who use processes which involve as little heat and light as possible. In such situations, sometimes going old school and traditional might be better than any newfangled methods.

The key is to look out for the absence of heat, and light, as well as pressure, in the extraction method for the fish oil. Absence of chemical additives is also a big plus in ensuring you get organic, non-contaminated fish oil. It might seem a tall order, and I would have to say it is from no small amount of research on my part that I discovered this particular brand of fish oil which happened to be extracted in the traditional Viking manner, excluding modern impediments like light, heat, pressure and chemical additives. Just type "Rosita fish oil" into any search engine and you should be able to get to the company's website.

I would like to state here that this is what I use personally, and I have seen good results from sustained consumption of their extra virgin cod liver oil. I am by no means affiliated to the company nor am I endorsing it. This is just something I would like to share with anyone who is looking for quality fish oil supplements in a bid to boost their omega-3 intake. Omega-3 fatty acids are crucial for brain health, and studies have shown that patients who suffered from traumatic brain injuries saw enhanced recovery when eicosapentaenoic acid (EPA) and docosahexaenoic acid (DHA), two of the more prominent omega-3 acids, were directly introduced via the intravenous system. Omega-3 acids are also important in regulating the body's inflammatory response. Their presence produces anti-inflammatory substances which goes a long way in balancing out the harmful effects of sugar and trans fats present in the modern diet.

Omega-6 acids are necessary for proper inflammatory function as well, since they contain triggers which sets off the inflammation reaction in the body. A proper inflammatory response is needed in the body to act as a kind of firewall or defense against foreign pathogens and harmful substances that may otherwise hurt us. The key here is the balance between omega-3 and -6 acids, where the optimal ratio is seen as two parts omega-3 to one part omega-6. You want to be able to rally your body's defense forces when enemies appear at the gates, but in the same context, you also want to be able to stand them down after the viruses are squashed. Having the body's defense keyed up for too long is a perfect recipe for chronic inflammation.

The final kind of fat that we are looking at would be saturated fat. This is where the more serious debates and arguments would take place pertaining to the impact that this fat has on human health. Some staunch believers of the theory that connects saturated fat to heart disease still hold out that cutting down on saturated fat would dramatically help lower cholesterol as well as the risks of cardiovascular disease. Others, however, point to increasing evidence that saturated fat has no bearing on the development of heart disease. Saturated fat gets its bad reputation for heart problems due to the fact that it is thought to clog up arteries through the formation of atherosclerotic plaque. The plaque comprises of fat and cholesterol, as well as other substances, and it does make for a very viable case to state that fat is primarily responsible for the formation of this life-threatening plaque. Except that things aren't always what they seem.

If we delve a little deeper into the function of atherosclerotic plaque, the easy theory of saturated fats clogging arteries, like waste jamming up the kitchen sink and pipes, might seem a trifle flimsy. Think about it: if saturated fats were really that bad, folks in the era of our grandparents and great grandparents would have been subjects of a heart disease epidemic! They were consuming red meat, lard, cheeses and other full cream dairy products that were all high in saturated fat. Why is it that our forefathers found it alright to have these full fat foods without any major medical issues but we would be singing a different tune when consuming the same foods? The issue, it seems, lies not with fats, but with our modern obsession with sugar.

Sugar has been rightfully identified as one of the main causes of chronic inflammation and the primary culprit for quite a number of debilitating ailments that seem to flourish in the developed world. Diabetes, Alzheimer's, and even metabolic syndrome have all been attributed in whole or in part to the elevated presence of sugar in our modern diet. As it happens, inflammation also occurs in our organs and arteries, and our bodies, being this amazing biochemical supercomputer, will then deploy healing substances to those inflamed areas in a bid to rectify or cordon off the problem. This is what happens in the case of our arteries, suffering and damaged from the sugar onslaught, the plaque that forms is created by our bodies to cover up the areas in distress and try to heal them. Picture a gash or a cut on your arm, as it is healing, a scab would form to protect the wound from re-opening, which is exactly what is happening with the formation of arterial plaque. The plaque forms in a bid to allow the body to heal the affected arteries. More often than not though, the body would still be subjected to high amounts of sugar through diet and healing is definitely impaired. When the area is rendered irreparable, the body then attempts to shield this damaged portion away from the rest of the healthy system, and that is when atherosclerosis begins in earnest.

Some folks may still wonder about the levels of cholesterol and fat found in the arterial plaque and point to that as a source of concern. It might come as no surprise to know that cholesterol is one of the more important ingredients needed when the body has a need to heal itself. This is why cholesterol is listed as an essential substance for the human body. There are many who are concerned with high cholesterol readings, but low cholesterol levels are also a cause for medical concern, because it implies a potential problem in the body's healing ability. Saturated fat also plays its role in ensuring proper nerve signaling as well as optimizing the immune system's performance. This immune system regulation becomes crucial when we are talking about healing processes in our body. With the presence of cholesterol and saturated fat in arterial plaque explained, I would surmise that this should set most minds at ease about saturated fat! Remember, all types of fat are required by the body for essential function, so it would really be counterproductive for a diet to espouse low fat. Remember, the brain is made of mostly saturated fats, and saturated fats are needed for it to maintain optimal function. The myelin sheath, an insulating substance for proper nerve transmissions and signaling, counts cholesterol and fat as its more important formative components. Saturated fat foods would be a source of ample supply for these building blocks.

At this juncture, we know that fat is needed and is, in fact, a necessary ingredient in many of the important body processes required to sustain life. Also, we could probably do ourselves a favor and banish the link between healthy, organic fats and cardiovascular disease. Note that I said healthy and organic fats. Trans fats or franken fats still should remain on the top of your watch list for banned substances! So go ahead and enjoy the healthy full fat foods you find aplenty in the ketogenic diet with a peace of mind, because this is a great chance to get the body back into an optimal metabolic state and turn it into a natural fat burning machine to boot!

Ketosis Versus Ketoacidosis

Whenever I am in the initial stage of helping a friend ease into the keto diet or just plainly getting to know more about it, I am almost always certain that this question on ketoacidosis will crop up, so I thought it might be useful to include this section to clear the air on this.

Ketoacidosis is primarily a situation when the body has little or no insulin to ferry the glucose present in the blood stream back into cells for use or storage. The body then gets the impression it is starving and in need of energy, hence ketone production is activated in the liver to correct this issue. However, the body does not get the signal to slow or stop ketone production because there is insufficient insulin in the system to do this. Ketones then build up in the blood, together with glucose, and the elevated levels cause ketoacidosis.

Some of the symptoms of ketoacidosis would sound awfully familiar with nutritional ketosis.

- Many trips to the toilet for urination
- Feeling really thirsty all the time
- Experiencing constant vomiting
- Stomach pains as well as constant nausea
- Feeling tired and mentally confused
- Feeling of insufficient air or shortness of breath

Frequent urination as well as being tired and in a state of mental fatigue are also common occurrences when someone is going through the initial stages of ketosis. This is where the body is getting used to the low carb lifestyle and making its metabolic adjustments. Those symptoms may be annoying but are harmless, and more importantly, they will pass after the first few weeks of ketosis.

To be definitive in identifying ketoacidosis, the trick here is not to just zoom in on one particular symptom and become overly worried. Ketoacidosis symptoms usually present themselves together, and if you were to be forced to pick one particular symptom to pay attention to, that would be the constant vomiting. When that is present together with stomach pains and a shortness of breath, immediate medical treatment is needed as ketoacidosis can be a life threatening issue.

The key here is the insufficient supply or lack of insulin. This is a situation where most type 1 diabetic patients would find themselves, as well as, to a lesser extent, some type 2 diabetics. When the pancreas cannot produce the level of insulin needed to signal the halt of ketone production, that is when ketone levels can go into overdrive and induce overly acidic conditions in the blood.

This does not mean type 1 diabetics or folks who rely on external insulin sources cannot be following the ketogenic diet. They still can, on the condition that they monitor and maintain adequate insulin levels in the body. In cases where the pancreas is still in relatively good shape and able to supply adequate amounts of insulin, the keto diet will be able to effectively correct the insulin desensitivity of the body's cells and improve or even reverse type 2 diabetic conditions.

Other Good Stuff From The Ketogenic Lifestyle

More than just having the potential to reverse type 2 diabetes, the ketogenic diet has multiple beneficial effects which I have listed below. This will be a good motivational booster or reminder during instances along the keto journey when the going gets tough and throwing in the towel becomes a somewhat palatable option. Don't give up! These are the good things awaiting you at the end of the rainbow!

Natural hunger suppression – Like what has been elaborated previously, this feature of the keto diet comes in really handy when your goal is to achieve some weight loss. You can now do so without suffering from crazy hunger pangs.

Sustainable weight loss and maintenance – Another thing that has it going for the ketogenic diet is the fact that you practically do not have to watch out for any sudden weight rebounds or crazy weight gains if you keep on track with the diet. The mechanics of ketosis does not allow that to happen, and of course, we are talking about normal meals here, not seven or eight thousand calorie food plans which would definitely upset the weight loss process. You still can put on weight if you eat too much!

Clearer thoughts in the mind – Due to the neuroprotective benefits that ketones actually confer on the brain, one of the additional advantages of going keto would be experiencing a sharper and clearer mind. Thought processes are touched with more clarity, without the brain fog that is common for folks on processed carb-rich diets. Ketones burning more efficiently as fuel also contributes to this enhanced mental clarity.

Experience better and more stable moods – When the body enters ketosis, the ketones generated for energy also help with the balance between two neurotransmitters that govern the brain: GABA, also known as gamma-aminobutyric acid, as well as glutamate. GABA serves to calm the brain down, while glutamate acts as a stimulant for the cerebral system. The trick to a healthy and happy brain is to keep these two substances in correct balance, and ketones certainly help to achieve that end.

Improve energy levels and solve chronic fatigue – Instead of having roller coaster spikes in your energy levels, the ketone fueled body will allow you to experience increased energy levels that stay more or less constant as long as you have your meals when hunger hits. Chronic fatigue also becomes a non-issue due to the elevated levels of energy. Even if the chronic fatigue is a symptom of other diseases, many find that though it does not go away entirely, the tiredness gets better on the keto diet.

Get your inflammation levels down – When you ensure that you have the adequate balance of omega-3 fats, these healthy polyunsaturated fats help to decrease the inflammatory response in the body system. This makes for good news to those who are suffering from chronic inflammatory diseases. Besides, the carb restriction would probably see your sugar intake coming way down, which will definitely help in reducing inflammation as well.

Lower your triglycerides reading – With a reduced carb intake, the level of triglycerides in the blood would automatically be lowered. Triglycerides form when we have excess calories, usually from carbs, so that the body can begin the process of storing the unrequired energy as fats. When the body is fueled predominantly by ketones and not by glucose, the need for producing triglycerides actually reduces due to the change in dietary habit. On keto, you eat when you are really hungry, and not because of wildly fluctuating blood sugar levels as well as the siren call of carbs.

Improve your lipid panel readouts – Going keto will usually see your HDL cholesterol going up while the LDL cholesterol levels will go the other direction. There may be some instances where you will see both HDL and LDL levels increase, resulting in an overall increase in cholesterol levels. Some folks have expressed concern on this matter and I would like to elaborate a little more on this. LDL and total cholesterol levels may become elevated for some who go on the ketogenic diet, but this should not totally freak you out! Think of it in this manner: if your body has been damaged metabolically through the years of eating processed and sugary carbs, the increase in cholesterol is actually a sign that the body is going through a healing cycle in order to normalize metabolic function. When the damage is largely repaired, LDL and total cholesterol levels tend to start tilting downward. Everyone's body is different, and so too is the time taken for the repair to be effected. Some might see results in months, while others may need a year or two to get the optimal levels.

Less oxidative stress – The ketogenic diet is responsible for increasing the antioxidants present in the body, while also directly reducing the oxidation that is encountered by the body's mitochondria. With boosted antioxidant activity whilst on the keto diet, free radicals tend to have a harder time in inflicting oxidative damage on our bodies. Less oxidation usually means that our cells and organs function better and enjoy a longer shelf life. This also means that there could be a chance to prolong our longevity, since oxidation, being one of the prime reasons behind aging, sees its activity being restrained to some extent while on the ketogenic diet.

These are only some of the benefits which you will get to enjoy when you go keto. I would have loved to put in more information, especially where the ketogenic diet has had positive effects on diseases like cancer, polycystic ovary syndrome, non-alcoholic fatty liver disease, and neurodegenerative ailments like Parkinson's and Alzheimer's.

However, the intent of this book has always been to provide delicious and savory culinary solutions for the keto dieter. It might be a good idea to pop over to my other book, *Ketogenic Diet. The Step by Step Guide for Beginners: Optimal Path to Effective Weight Loss*, where I go into more details on the various benefits of the keto diet. In it, I also give an easy to follow, step by step road map which would definitely ease you into ketosis, as well as highlighting those nitty gritty bits of useful information to look out for. Definitely of value to the keto beginner, and also a handy book to have around as a reminder for the more seasoned keto dieter, you can pick your copy from the US or wherever you may be around the globe.

Chapter 2
The Yes And No Of Keto Foods

Now we are getting to the meat of things! This chapter is going to start by fleshing out the foods which you will be getting intimately acquainted with. Oh yes, the fatty meats as well as dairy products will feature, and don't forget your greens and fruits! There will be another section on what kind of foods to cut down on in order to limit your carb consumption. The lists are meant to act as a sort of easy primer when it comes to keto friendly foods, so that it becomes easier for you to pick out and identify which foods are good to go during meal times.

As we know, the standard ketogenic diet macronutrient requirements are as follows

- 75% Fats
- 20% Protein
- 5% Carbohydrates

When we translate this to a daily intake of 2,000 calories, that means we are looking at 1,500 calories from fats, 400 calories from protein and the remaining 100 calories from carbs. With each gram of protein and carb yielding 4 calories, and each gram of fat yielding 9 calories, the whole breakdown above will end up with a daily grand figure of approximately 166 grams of fat, 100 grams of protein and 25 grams of carbs. These macronutrient numbers should be at the forefront of your mind when you first start off with the ketogenic diet. Just remember, always try to hit your fat requirement, limit your carb intake, and think about the amount of protein you are getting in to your system.

If your experience is anything like mine, you will find that eating sufficient fat seems to be an issue, at least in the initial stages. This is partly because a lot of the fat that you take in is present in liquid forms. Think of olive and coconut oils, or the butter and lard when heated on the skillet, these are all high fat essentials in the keto diet but they can be easily overlooked because they will never be the mains in a meal. I found that keeping the count on my daily fat numbers helped in increasing my fat intake. On the days when you find the fat count being a little low, 99% dark chocolate as well as bulletproof coffee can nudge those numbers up closer to where they are supposed to be. Of course, there are many other high fat foods which can do the trick as well, so let's take a look at them!

Foods To Enjoy On The Ketogenic Diet

There are different types of food that fall into this list. These food ideas definitely push for high fat content, while at the same time packing other nutrients and healthy vitamins in for the body's use.

Meats And Animal Products – Focus on grass-fed or pasture-raised fatty cuts of meat and wild-caught seafood, avoiding farmed animal meats and processed meats as much as possible. And don't forget about organ meats!

- Beef
- Chicken
- Eggs
- Goat
- Lamb
- Pork
- Rabbit
- Turkey
- Venison
- Shellfish
- Salmon
- Mackerel
- Tuna
- Halibut
- Cod
- Gelatin
- Organ meats

Healthy Fats – The best fats to consume on the ketogenic diet are monounsaturated and polyunsaturated fats, though there are plenty of healthy saturated fats as well. At the risk of sounding like a broken recorder, avoid trans fats. Maybe "avoid" is not an appropriate word. Run away might be better. Run away from trans fats like you would the plague. Enough said.

- Butter
- Chicken fat
- Coconut oil
- Duck fat
- Ghee
- Lard
- Tallow
- MCT oil
- Avocado oil
- Macadamia oil
- Extra virgin olive oil
- Coconut butter
- Coconut milk
- Palm shortening

Vegetables – Fresh vegetables are rich in nutrients and low in calories which makes them an excellent addition to any diet. With the ketogenic diet, however, you need to be careful about carbs, so stick to leafy greens and low-glycemic veggies rather than root vegetables and other starchy veggies. I placed avocados in this section because some of us may recognize it as a vegetable even though it actually is a fruit.

- Artichokes
- Asparagus
- Avocado
- Bell peppers
- Broccoli
- Cabbage
- Cauliflower
- Cucumber
- Celery
- Kohlrabi
- Lettuce
- Okra or ladies' fingers
- Radishes
- Seaweed
- Spinach
- Tomatoes
- Watercress
- Zucchini

Dairy Products – If you are able to tolerate dairy, you can include full-fat, unpasteurized, and raw dairy products in your diet. Keep in mind that some brands will contain a lot of sugar which could increase the carb content, so pay attention to nutrition labels and moderate your consumption of these products. If possible, go for the full-fat versions as these will have a less likely chance of sugar being used to replace the fat.

- Kefir
- Cottage cheese
- Cream cheese
- Cheddar cheese
- Brie cheese
- Mozzarella cheese
- Swiss cheese
- Sour cream
- Full-fat yogurt
- Heavy cream

Herbs And Spices – Fresh herbs and dried spices are an excellent way to flavor your foods without adding any significant number of calories or carbohydrates

- Basil
- Black pepper
- Cayenne
- Cardamom
- Chili powder
- Cilantro
- Cinnamon
- Cumin
- Curry powder
- Garam masala
- Ginger
- Garlic
- Nutmeg
- Oregano
- Onion
- Paprika
- Parsley
- Rosemary
- Sea salt
- Sage
- Thyme
- Turmeric
- White pepper

Beverages – You should avoid all sweetened drinks on the ketogenic diet, but there are certain beverages which you can still have in order to add a little more variety to your choice of liquids besides good old water.

- Almond milk unsweetened
- Bone broth
- Cashew milk unsweetened
- Coconut milk
- Club soda
- Coffee
- Herbal tea
- Mineral water
- Seltzer water
- Tea

Foods On The Moderation List

These food items are included here because they tend to have a higher carb count, so moderation is important. However, they are chock full of other nutrients and some of them also throw in that extra bit of fat to help toward your daily fat intake!

Fruits – Fresh fruits are an excellent source of nutrition. Unfortunately, they are also loaded with sugar which means they are high in carbohydrates. There are a few low- to moderate-carb fruits that you can enjoy in smaller quantities, but you have to watch the amount you eat! Sometimes, it is really easy to keep popping them into our mouths. "Nature's candy" is definitely an accurate moniker for them. We can still get their benefits and maintain ketosis with the right amounts of consumption. Most of the fruits detailed below are okay for you to have a cup or so, perhaps a single slice or two on a daily basis, especially when you are first starting out and are looking to keep your carb count low. As you progress and get a better handle of your carb threshold, it is alright to increase the quantity of these foods while staying within your designated carb limit.

- Apricot
- Blackberries
- Blueberries
- Cantaloupe
- Cherries
- Cranberries
- Grapefruit
- Honeydew
- Kiwi
- Lemon
- Lime
- Peaches
- Raspberries
- Strawberries

Nuts And Seeds – While nuts and seeds do contain carbohydrates, they are also rich in healthy fats. The following nuts and seeds are low to moderate in carb content, so you can enjoy them as long as you watch your portion sizes. Usually an ounce or a handful of nuts would be a good gauge to see how much you can eat and still stay in ketosis daily.

- Almonds
- Cashews
- Chia seeds
- Hazelnuts
- Macadamia nuts
- Pecans
- Pine nuts
- Pistachios
- Psyllium
- Pumpkin seeds
- Sesame seeds
- Sunflower seeds
- Walnuts
- Nut butter

Foods To Avoid

When it comes to foods you should avoid on the ketogenic diet, there are a few major categories to mention. First and foremost, you should avoid grains and grain-based ingredients as much as possible since they are the highest in carbohydrates. Choose healthy fats over hydrogenated oils and try to limit your intake of starchy vegetables and high-glycemic fruits. When it comes to sweeteners, refined sugars like white sugar and brown sugar are completely restricted, and you should also avoid artificial sweeteners. Natural sweeteners like honey, pure maple syrup, and agave are not necessarily bad for you, but they are very high in carbohydrates. The best sweeteners to use on the ketogenic diet are powdered erythritol, stevia, and monk fruit sweetener.

Stevia is an herb that is also known as the sugar leaf. This sweetener comes in several forms, and you need to make sure that whatever type you buy doesn't also contain an artificial sweetener. Liquid stevia extract is usually the best option, though you can also find powdered stevia extract. Another option is powdered erythritol, which is extracted from corn, and it is usually the best option to use in recipes for baked goods. In terms of sauces and condiments, you need to read the food label to see whether the item is keto-friendly or not because brands differ greatly. Generally speaking, basic condiments like yellow mustard, mayonnaise, horseradish, hot sauce, Worcestershire sauce, vinegar, and oils are keto-friendly. When it comes to things like ketchup, BBQ sauce, and salad dressings you need to be mindful of the sugar content present in them.

Here is a quick list of some of the major foods you'll need to avoid on the ketogenic diet.

- All-purpose flour
- Baking mix
- Wheat flour
- Pastry flour
- Cake flour
- Cereal
- Pasta
- Rice
- Corn
- Baked goods
- Corn syrup
- Snack bars
- Quinoa
- Buckwheat
- Barley
- Couscous
- Oats
- Muesli
- Margarine
- Canola oil
- Hydrogenated oils
- Bananas
- Mangos
- Pineapple
- Potatoes
- Sweet potatoes
- Candy
- Milk chocolate
- Ice cream
- Sports drinks
- Juice cocktail
- Soda
- Beer
- Milk
- Low-fat dairy
- White sugar
- Brown sugar
- Maple syrup
- Honey
- Agave

What To Look Out For In Some Keto Foods

Since this is very much serving as a recipe book, I thought it would be appropriate to share some tips and ideas on what to look out for when we are choosing the more common and popular keto foods for prepping our meals.

Salmon – This fatty fish has always ranked high for me when it comes to keto friendly foods. You may know it to be packed with beneficial omega-3 polyunsaturated fats, which boost brain health and help with reducing inflammation, but it also has loads of other nutrients which the body needs.

Potassium and selenium are found in bountiful amounts when it comes to salmon. Potassium is integral to proper regulation of blood pressure as well as the body's water retention. Selenium helps out with maintaining good bone health as well as ensuring an optimal immune system. On top of this, salmon also contains healthy levels of B vitamins. These vitamins are crucial for efficient food to energy processing, as well as maintaining the proper function of both the body's DNA and nervous system. To top it off, salmon has astaxanthin, an antioxidant which gives salmon flesh its reddish-pink hue. This powerful antioxidant helps with heart and brain health, and may also be beneficial for the skin.

To get a good quality deal, the first thing you should take note of is the smell. Fresh salmon, or any fish for that matter, will not really have an odor. You can probably smell a tinge of the ocean, but fresh fish will definitely not smell fishy. When it is fishy, you know that fish is not for you.

Next up, pay attention to the eyes. Look for those with clear and shiny eyes. Think of a movie star who has teared up - those are the kind of eyes that best demonstrate what you are looking for. Never go for sunken or dry-looking eyes. Cloudy-looking ones are also a no-go when it comes to fresh fish selection.

Fins and gills are also areas which we want to pay attention to. Fresh fish have fins which look wet and whole, not torn and ragged. Their gills are bright red and clean, not brownish-red and slimy. Lastly, if you are allowed to, try pressing the flesh and seeing if it bounces back like how your own does. Flesh which is depressed and stays depressed should not end up in your kitchen.

For fillet cuts, the best you can do is pay attention to the color as well as how the piece looks. The color should be vibrant and bright. Varied hues ranging from red to coral to pink are acceptable, but always remember that the main thing is the brightness of the flesh. Next would be to spot any breaks or cracks in the flesh itself. These are indications that the fillet has been kept for some time and is no longer as fresh. Also, any pooling of water should also trigger alarm bells, because it means that the flesh structure has started to break down, and it is time to move on to another piece.

Pork belly – This is another probable staple in the keto diet. I've talked about it in my other book but here I want to concentrate on helping you choose a good cut for prepping your meals. Every 100 grams of pork belly contains about 50 grams of fat. Packing another 9 grams of protein and absolutely no carbs, you can be sure that this is a good food item to boost your daily fat count. On top of that, it can be absolutely easy to prepare delicious meals with it.

When choosing pork belly, you should look at the color of the cut. Go for the cuts that are reddish pink to darkish red. Meat which is lighter in color generally means the freshness may have faded. Greying or discoloration will definitely mean that decay has already set in and the meat should not be picked up.

The other thing you want to look for is the streaky white strips of fat present in the pork belly. Generally the more streaks it has, the better the marbling will be and that is good news for you. Always ensure that the marbling is white, because any yellow or greyish coloring would represent meat that has probably passed its sell-by date.

Avocado oil – I must be honest here and say that this oil, for me, has been a later stage addition when compared to olive and coconut oil. Extra virgin olive oil, as well as the versatile coconut oil have their rightful places in the pantheon of staple keto foods, but avocado oil might be giving them a run for their money.

Avocado oil for one, consists of mostly monounsaturated fat. This particular quirk ties in to a very important point. The oil is considered far more stable than any of its polyunsaturated fat cousins, like vegetable oil and even extra virgin olive oil. Besides that, avocado oil is known to have a higher smoke point, somewhere around 500 degrees Fahrenheit, than most vegetable oils. This makes it a valuable addition to the kitchen because the oil has a higher resistance to degeneration by heat. Add on the fact that it packs a healthy punch in terms of vitamins, minerals, phytochemicals, and antioxidants, you will realize that this is one oil you can potentially use for many different applications.

Some folks use it for hair and skin care, where the vitamin E rich oil is known to be easily absorbed without additional chemicals or other potentially harmful additives. Adding the oil into salads, vegetables, or fruits is also a great way to boost monounsaturated fat intake with very little inconvenience. You might even want to try drinking it raw, though it doesn't work for me as I found it to be a little too raw. Mixing it up with some lime or garlic has always been what I prefer.

Now let's talk a little on how to go about choosing the avocado oil. First up, we want to look at the source or origin of the oil, which typically means we need to know where and how the avocados were grown. In this respect, you need to look for a certified organic label to know that the avocados were grown without any synthetic additives. This ensures that the oil derived from the avocados do not contain any substances that could be detrimental to your health.

Next, we need to look at how the oil is extracted. Mechanical and chemical extraction methods used usually involves increased heat as well as potent chemicals to force out the oil from the mashed avocado pulp. The downside of this is that the heat and chemicals may reduce the beneficial nutrients and vitamins present in the oil. To address this, cold pressing, which is known as the least destructive method out there, ensures that the color, smell, and taste are as close to the original fruit as possible. You get better quality oil, and in addition to that, enjoy more nutrients.

The last item we need to look at is how the oil is refined, or not. Seriously, for best results, cold pressed oil that is unrefined and gotten from certified organic avocados, would rank amongst the top tiers, if not the top. The downside is that the shelf life is short, and the oil smells very... avocado-ish. That shouldn't be a problem if you use it often, and you should, considering the health benefits and convenience that it brings. The next best thing would be to have the oil naturally refined, where the manufacturers typically do straining and filtering in order to extend the shelf life. Always remember, the more the oil is refined, the less nutrition it will provide.

Before I forget, always opt for oils in dark-colored glass bottles or tins. This is a little similar to extra virgin olive oil where the oil can go rancid in the presence of heat and light. For avocado oil, though the majority of fats present consist of the monounsaturated variety, there still is a minor percentage of polyunsaturated fats. Hence, better to err on the side of caution and go for dark-colored glass bottles.

Ghee – This substance has been around since the Ayurvedic times, and it has always been listed as the cooking medium of choice. Ghee is clarified butter, which means butter that has been heated and is free of lactose as well as other milk solids. This also results in a higher smoke point compared to butter. It can go as high as 480 degrees Fahrenheit, that means you can really deep fry or roast without the risk of oxidation which releases harmful free radicals.

Removal of the lactose is great news for those who are lactose intolerant, yet still wish to partake in the nutty and rich flavor that comes with butter. Ghee can be a great alternative, and the taste might even be more flavorful. Packed with multiple fat soluble vitamins, it also contains short chain fatty acids which boost cardiovascular health as well as help fight inflammation. Ghee also has the distinct advantage of being able to last about three to four weeks at room temperature while it can keep for up to six months when refrigerated.

Ghee can definitely be found in most grocery stores. Check for it in the oil section, although some places may have it in the dairy portion. As with butter, you can always try to go for grass-fed varieties first to improve the nutrient intake and reduce the chance of having potential additives or chemicals mixed in. For me, I usually go for ghee packed either in tins or glass jars.

Lard – Lard is fat from pigs. Once vilified together with all the other saturated fat food sources, lard is enjoying a well-justified comeback! Every 100 grams of lard gives you about 30 grams of saturated fat, with polyunsaturated fat making up 10 grams and the monounsaturated variety yielding about 40 grams. No, there is no mistake. You are reading it correctly. Lard actually has more monounsaturated fat than saturated fat content. Little wonder why folks from the earlier generations really swore by lard and practically used it for most stuff involving cooking and baking.

Now that we modern folk are coming round to lard once again, it has been found to be one of the richer sources of vitamin D foods. You don't need to get all your vitamin D from the sun or fish, lard is also a tasty alternative! On top of that, lard is also good for high heat cooking because of its higher smoke point which stands around 375 degrees Fahrenheit. There is also less chance of rancidity or free radical production due to the presence of saturated fat content which gives lard that extra layer of fat stability. Did I already mention that lard tastes great as well? That is a point worth repeating, because there is just something about animal fat that gives food a really rich and flavorful texture.

Unfortunately, lard being sold in supermarkets and most stores aren't really good because they have probably undergone some form of hydrogenation in order to prolong shelf life. Prolonging supermarket lard's shelf life comes at the expense of our own if we choose to add it into our meals. You really should be looking to get high quality lard from your butcher or meat grocer. Good lard, also known as leaf lard, is derived from visceral fat around the kidneys and loin area of the pig. If that has run out, you can go for the next best alternative, which is lard that is slightly more solid and is derived from between the back skin and muscle. Untreated or unrefined lard must always be refrigerated to maintain its freshness.

Bell peppers – These colorful vegetables not only add in color and a crunchy bite to our daily meals but they also pack quite a healthy punch in the nutrients department. Rich in vitamins A and C, as well as providing us with folate and vitamin K for added good measure, bell peppers help with boosting our immune system and maintaining tissue health. The antioxidant lycopene, a kind of carotenoid that gives the peppers its color, is also responsible in helping to reduce inflammation, as well as being an active scavenger for the body's free radicals. It is also extremely versatile, being perfectly suitable to serve raw or lightly grilled. More good news? The carb count for 100 grams of bell peppers stand at a measly 5 grams, of which 2 grams consist of dietary fiber. We'll touch more on this subject of dietary fiber and how it impacts the carb count, but for now, just know that bell peppers have an intensely low carb count for all the nutritious goodness it packs.

The trick to choosing a bell pepper that you would want to have on your dinner table is easy - really. Go for the ones with bright, vivid colors. The ones with lighter colors may indicate they aren't that ripe yet.

Any with bruises and discoloration should be set aside and replaced with those which have a glossy sheen. Gently squeeze the vegetable to feel for tightness of the skin. One more thing to note is that a ripe bell pepper will actually feel heavier than it looks. This is because it has not suffered from moisture loss associated with over ripeness. Bell peppers can be stored in the refrigerator for up to 10 days, so be sure to pop them into the chill box once you bring them back from your grocery run.

The list above is meant to give some help when it comes to the physical selection of these foods mentioned. I am pretty sure you would like to keep quality and fresh foods around in your kitchen and I hope this section would have gone some distance in helping you do that on a consistent basis.

Next up, we will be covering the 28-day meal plan that has been artfully prepared for you. Starting off with easy recipes to let anyone get accustomed to the keto lifestyle, it progresses in variety over the weeks so that you do not get bored with having the same meals over and over again. Let's step up and take a look at what we have for you!

Chapter 3
A Keto Helper: The 28 Day Meal Plan

Now, the moment you've been waiting for – the meal plan!

In this chapter, you'll find a 28-day meal plan for the standard ketogenic diet, divided into four weeks. Every day you'll follow the plan to eat breakfast, lunch, and dinner, as well as a snack or dessert with a calorie range between 1,800 and 2,000.

One thing I want to mention before you get started is net carbs.

Many people who follow the ketogenic diet prefer to track net carbs rather than total carbs. To calculate net carbs, you simply take the total carb count of the meal and subtract the grams of fiber since fiber cannot be digested. Personally, I prefer to track total carbs like what I have mentioned in my first book, but I have included the grams of fiber and net carbs in these recipes, so you can choose which way to go.

Personally, I prefer more buffer when it comes to the carb count, because I want to reduce the number of obstacles keeping me from ketosis. Many of my readers as well as friends have raised this point and you can be sure quite a few nights or afternoons were spent in heated debate! Okay, it wasn't that serious but suffice it to say that quite a bit of discussion went into this topic. Therefore, I thought it might be better if I gave you a say in this net carb-total carb debate. You get to choose whichever you prefer. In my personal opinion, when you are in the initial stages of trying to enter ketosis, keeping your total carb count in mind is probably one of the better practices you can adopt. A 20 to 50 gram range of carbs would usually work to push the body into a ketogenic state.

After you have gotten keto adapted and the body gets used to burning fat for fuel, you can then start to bring net carbs into the equation.

Keep in mind the calorie range for these meal plans – if you read my first book and calculated your own daily caloric needs, you may need to make some adjustments. If you're trying the ketogenic diet for the first time, however, it may be easiest to just follow the plan as is until you get the hang of it.

The first week of this 28-day meal plan is designed to be incredibly simple in terms of meal prep so you can focus on learning which foods to eat and which to avoid on the ketogenic diet – that's why you'll find more smoothies and soups here than in the following weeks. If you finish the first week and feel like you still need some time making the adjustment to keto, feel free to repeat it before moving on to week two. The meal plans also take into account left-overs and the yields of various recipes, so that you have minimal waste from your efforts in the kitchen.

So, without further ado, let's take a look at the meal plans!

Standard Keto Meal Plan - Week 1

Day	Breakfast	Lunch	Dinner	Snack/Dessert	Calories/Macros
1	Sheet Pan Eggs with Veggies and Parmesan with 6 oz Sliced Ham	Cucumber Avocado Salad with Bacon	Grilled Pesto Salmon with Asparagus and 2 Slices Thick-Cut Bacon	Pumpkin Spiced Almonds and (2) Coco-Macadamia Fat Bombs	Calories: 1940 Fat: 144.5g Protein: 113g Net Carbs: 21.5g
2	Kale Avocado Smoothie with 3 Slices Thick-Cut Bacon	Bacon Cheeseburger Soup	Leftover Grilled Pesto Salmon with Asparagus and 3 Slices Thick-Cut Bacon	Tzatziki Dip with Cauliflower and (1) Coco-Macadamia Fat Bomb	Calories: 1845 Fat: 140.5g Protein: 116g Net Carbs: 28.5g
3	Leftover Sheet Pan Eggs with Veggies and Parmesan and 3 Slices Thick-Cut Bacon	Leftover Bacon Cheeseburger Soup	Cheddar-Stuffed Burgers with Zucchini and ½ Cup Avocado	Pumpkin Spiced Almonds and (1) Coco-Macadamia Fat Bomb	Calories: 1875 Fat: 142.5g Protein: 123.5g Net Carbs: 22g
4	Almond Butter Protein Smoothie with 1 Cup Avocado	Ham and Provolone Sandwich	Chicken Cordon Bleu with Cauliflower and ½ Cup Avocado	Tzatziki Dip with Cauliflower and (1) Coco-Macadamia Fat Bomb	Calories: 1990 Fat: 149.5g Protein: 118.5g Net Carbs: 31g
5	Leftover Sheet Pan Eggs with Veggies and Parmesan and 2 Slices Thick-Cut Bacon	Leftover Bacon Cheeseburger Soup	Leftover Cheddar-Stuffed Burgers with Zucchini	Pumpkin Spiced Almonds and (2) Coco-Macadamia Fat Bombs	Calories: 1880 Fat: 146g Protein: 118.5g Net Carbs: 23.5g
6	Beets and Blueberry Smoothie with 2 Slices Thick-Cut Bacon	Baked Chicken Nuggets	Leftover Chicken Cordon Bleu with Cauliflower and 1 Cup Avocado	Tzatziki Dip with Cauliflower and (1) Coco-Macadamia Fat Bomb	Calories: 1915 Fat: 147g Protein: 114g Net Carbs: 27.5g
7	Leftover Sheet Pan Eggs with Veggies and Parmesan and 3 Slices Thick-Cut Bacon	Taco Salad with Creamy Dressing	Leftover Chicken Cordon Bleu with Cauliflower and ½ Cup Avocado	Pumpkin Spiced Almonds and (1) Coco-Macadamia Fat Bomb	Calories: 1980 Fat: 152.5g Protein: 122.5g Net Carbs: 24.5g

\underline{Day}	\underline{Breakfast}	\underline{Lunch}	\underline{Dinner}	\underline{Snack/Dessert}	\underline{Calories/Macros}
	Standard Keto Meal Plan - Week 2				
8	Almond Butter Muffin with 6 oz Sliced Ham	Egg Salad Over Lettuce with 2 Slices Thick-Cut Bacon	Sesame-Crusted Tuna with Green Beans	Curry-Roasted Macadamia Nuts and (2) Sesame Almond Fat Bombs	Calories: 1940 Fat: 155g Protein: 112.5g Net Carbs: 21
9	Classic Western Omelet	Egg Drop Soup with 3 Slices Thick-Cut Bacon	Leftover Sesame-Crusted Tuna with Green Beans and ½ Cup Avocado	Overnight Coconut Chia Pudding and (1) Sesame Almond Fat Bomb	Calories: 1970 Fat: 152.5g Protein: 118g Net Carbs: 24.5g
10	Almond Butter Muffin with 6 oz Sliced Ham	Leftover Egg Drop Soup with 3 Slices Thick-Cut Bacon	Rosemary Roasted Pork with Cauliflower and 1 Cup Avocado	Curry-Roasted Macadamia Nuts and (1) Sesame Almond Fat Bomb	Calories: 1905 Fat: 148.5g Protein: 17g Net Carbs: 16g
11	Cinnamon Protein Pancakes	Bacon, Lettuce, Tomato, Avocado Sandwich with 5 oz Sliced Ham	Chicken Tikka with Cauliflower Rice	Overnight Coconut Chia Pudding and (1) Sesame Almond Fat Bomb	Calories: 1990 Fat: 158.5g Protein: 114g Net Carbs: 20.5g
12	Almond Butter Muffin with 6 oz Sliced Ham	Leftover Egg Drop Soup with 3 Slices Thick-Cut Bacon	Leftover Rosemary Roasted Pork with Cauliflower and 1 Cup Avocado	Curry-Roasted Macadamia Nuts and (1) Sesame Almond Fat Bombs	Calories: 1905 Fat: 148.5g Protein: 117g Net Carbs: 16g
13	Cinnamon Protein Pancakes	Fried Salmon Cakes	Leftover Rosemary Roasted Pork with Cauliflower and 4 oz Sliced Ham	Overnight Coconut Chia Pudding and (1) Sesame Almond Fat Bomb	Calories: 1925 Fat: 148.5g Protein: 118g Net Carbs: 20.5g
14	Almond Butter Muffin with 6 oz Sliced Ham	Spring Salad with Shaved Parmesan and 3 Slices Thick-Cut Bacon	Leftover Chicken Tikka with Cauliflower Rice	Curry-Roasted Macadamia Nuts and (1) Sesame Almond Fat Bomb	Calories: 1920 Fat: 152g Protein: 118.5g Net Carbs: 17.5g

Standard Keto Meal Plan - Week 3

Day	Breakfast	Lunch	Dinner	Snack/Dessert	Calories/Macros
15	Sheet Pan Eggs with Ham and Pepper Jack and 6 oz. Sliced Ham	Sesame Chicken Avocado Salad	Grilled Salmon and Zucchini with Mango Sauce	Chocolate Almond Butter Brownie and (2) Layered Almond Chocolate Fat Bombs	Calories: 1825 Fat: 144g Protein: 114g Net Carbs: 17.5g
16	Detoxifying Green Smoothie with 4 Slices Thick-Cut Bacon	Spinach Cauliflower Soup with 4 Slices Thick-Cut Bacon	Leftover Grilled Salmon and Zucchini with Mango Sauce	Bacon Cheeseburger Bites and (1) Layered Almond Chocolate Fat Bomb	Calories: 1850 Fat: 139.5g Protein: 125.5g Net Carbs: 25
17	Leftover Sheet Pan Eggs with Ham and Pepper Jack and 4 Slices Thick-Cut Bacon	Leftover Spinach Cauliflower Soup with 1 Medium Avocado	Slow-Cooker Pot Roast with Green Beans	Chocolate Almond Butter Brownie and (1) Layered Almond Chocolate Fat Bomb	Calories: 1940 Fat: 150g Protein: 117.5g Net Carbs: 21g
18	Nutty Pumpkin Smoothie with 1 Cup Avocado	Cheesy Buffalo Chicken Sandwich	Beef and Broccoli Stir-Fry with ½ Cup Avocado	Bacon Cheeseburger Bites and (1) Layered Almond Chocolate Fat Bomb	Calories: 1935 Fat: 139.5g Protein: 130g Net Carbs: 24.5g
19	Leftover Sheet Pan Eggs with Ham and Pepper Jack and 1 Medium Avocado	Leftover Spinach Cauliflower Soup with 3 Slices Thick-Cut Bacon	Leftover Slow-Cooker Pot Roast with Green Beans	Chocolate Almond Butter Brownie and (1) Layered Almond Chocolate Fat Bomb	Calories: 1840 Fat: 142g Protein: 111.5g Net Carbs: 20.5g
20	Vanilla Chai Smoothie with 1 Cup Avocado	Coconut Chicken Tenders with 1 Cup Avocado	Leftover Slow-Cooker Pot Roast with Green Beans	Bacon Cheeseburger Bites and (1) Layered Almond Chocolate Fat Bomb	Calories: 2005 Fat: 139g Protein: 147g Net Carbs: 16g
21	Leftover Sheet Pan Eggs with Ham and Pepper Jack and 6 oz. Sliced Ham	Avocado Spinach Salad with Almonds and 3 Slices Thick-Cut Bacon	Leftover Beef and Broccoli Stir-Fry	Chocolate Almond Butter Brownie and (1) Layered Almond Chocolate Fat Bomb	Calories: 1840 Fat: 141.5g Protein: 118.5g Net Carbs: 16.5g

Standard Keto Meal Plan - Week 4

Day	Breakfast	Lunch	Dinner	Snack/Dessert	Calories/Macros
22	Tomato Mozzarella Egg Muffins with 6 oz. Sliced Ham	Easy Chopped Salad	Parmesan-Crusted Halibut with Asparagus and 1 Medium Avocado	Coconut Vanilla Cupcake and (1) Layered Coco-Chia Fat Bomb	Calories: 1980 Fat: 150g Protein: 116g Net Carbs: 21g
23	Crispy Chai Waffles with 6 oz. Sliced Ham	Cauliflower Leek Soup with Pancetta and 3 Slices Thick-Cut Bacon	Leftover Parmesan-Crusted Halibut with Asparagus and 1 Cup Avocado	Cinnamon Quick Bread and (1) Layered Coco-Chia Fat Bomb	Calories: 1985 Fat: 148g Protein: 119.5g Net Carbs: 23g
24	Leftover Tomato Mozzarella Egg Muffins with 6 oz. Sliced Ham	Leftover Cauliflower Leek Soup with Pancetta and 3 Slices Thick-Cut Bacon	Hearty Beef and Bacon Casserole	Coconut Vanilla Cupcake and (2) Layered Coco-Chia Fat Bombs	Calories: 1980 Fat: 150g Protein: 117g Net Carbs: 23g
25	Leftover Crispy Chai Waffles with 6 oz Sliced Ham	Three Meat and Cheese Sandwich	Sesame Wings with Cauliflower and ½ Cup Avocado	Cinnamon Quick Bread and (1) Layered Coco-Chia Fat Bomb	Calories: 1930 Fat: 147g Protein: 114g Net Carbs: 16.5g
26	Leftover Tomato Mozzarella Egg Muffins with 6 oz. Sliced Ham	Leftover Cauliflower Leek Soup with Pancetta and 4 Slices Thick-Cut Bacon	Leftover Hearty Beef and Bacon Casserole with 1 Cup Avocado	Coconut Vanilla Cupcake and (1) Layered Coco-Chia Fat Bomb	Calories: 1950 Fat: 143.5g Protein: 122g Net Carbs: 22g
27	Broccoli Kale Egg Scramble with 2 Slices Thick-Cut Bacon	Beef and Pepper Kebabs	Leftover Hearty Beef and Bacon Casserole with 1 Cup Avocado	Cinnamon Quick Bread and (1) Layered Coco-Chia Fat Bomb	Calories: 1965 Fat: 148g Protein: 115.5g Net Carbs: 27g
28	Leftover Tomato Mozzarella Egg Muffins with 6 oz. Sliced Ham	Simple Tuna Salad on Lettuce	Leftover Sesame Wings with Cauliflower and ½ Cup Avocado	Coconut Vanilla Cupcake and (1) Layered Coco-Chia Fat Bomb	Calories: 1960 Fat: 148g Protein: 123.5g Net Carbs: 20g

Chapter 4
Step By Step: High Fat Low Carb Keto Recipes

This chapter is all about the recipes! Step by step instructions on how to prepare them and get these delicious foods from the kitchen onto your dining plates. Just a wee bit of a hold up here, before we dive into these recipes, I thought this additional gift would be of some value to you.

An Additional Gift Of Recipe Cards. You can download them from this web link www.fcmediapublishing.com/recipecardsjkm2

You can download it by going to the link above. What is it? It's a collection of 30 recipes from this cookbook which I thought would be useful to collate into handy recipe card formats. Call it culinary visual motivation if you will, because all 30 recipes come with hi-res images of the foods which you are about to prepare. You can print it out, laminate them and have them lying around for useful reference in the kitchen without any fear of damage.

That's it! No muss, no fuss, to get your 30 recipe cards which you can put to good use by having both the cooking instructions and the pictures of the finished article right in front of you.

To make it simpler, all recipes are categorized into breakfast, lunch, and dinner, as well as desserts and snack bombs.

Breakfast Recipes

- Sheet Pan Eggs with Veggies and Parmesan
- Kale Avocado Smoothie
- Almond Butter Protein Smoothie
- Beets and Blueberry Smoothie
- Almond Butter Muffins
- Classic Western Omelet
- Cinnamon Protein Pancakes
- Sheet Pan Eggs with Ham and Pepper Jack
- Detoxifying Green Smoothie
- Nutty Pumpkin Smoothie
- Tomato Mozzarella Egg Muffins
- Crispy Chai Waffles
- Broccoli Kale Egg Scramble
- Creamy Chocolate Protein Smoothie
- Three Cheese Egg Muffins
- Strawberry Rhubarb Pie Smoothie
- Vanilla Chai Smoothie
- Cinnamon Almond Porridge
- Bacon, Mushroom, and Swiss Omelet
- Maple Cranberry Muffins

- Coco-Cashew Macadamia Muffins
- Chocolate Protein Pancakes
- Ham, Cheddar, and Chive Omelet
- Spinach Parmesan Egg Scramble
- Cinnamon Roll Waffles
- Bacon Swiss Waffles
- Meaty Breakfast Omelet
- Lemon Flaxseed Muffins
- Pumpkin Spice Waffles

Lunch Recipes

- Cucumber Avocado Salad with Bacon
- Bacon Cheeseburger Soup
- Ham and Provolone Sandwich
- Baked Chicken Nuggets
- Taco Salad with Creamy Dressing
- Egg Salad Over Lettuce
- Egg Drop Soup
- Bacon, Lettuce, Tomato, Avocado Sandwich
- Fried Salmon Cakes
- Spring Salad with Shaved Parmesan
- Sesame Chicken Avocado Salad
- Spinach Cauliflower Soup
- Cheesy Buffalo Chicken Sandwich
- Coconut Chicken Tenders
- Avocado Spinach Salad with Almonds
- Easy Chopped Salad
- Cauliflower Leek Soup with Pancetta
- Three Meat and Cheese Sandwich
- Beef and Pepper Kebabs
- Simple Tuna Salad on Lettuce
- Ham, Egg, and Cheese Sandwich
- Bacon-Wrapped Hot Dogs
- Fried Tuna Avocado Balls
- Curried Chicken Soup
- Chopped Kale Salad with Bacon Dressing
- Kale Caesar Salad with Chicken
- Chicken Enchilada Soup
- Thai Coconut Shrimp Soup
- Mushroom and Asparagus Soup
- Slow-Cooker Chicken Fajita Soup
- Avocado Egg Salad on Lettuce

- Bacon-Wrapped Chicken Rolls
- Spicy Shrimp and Sausage Soup
- Slow-Cooker Beef Chili

Dinner Recipes

- Grilled Pesto Salmon with Asparagus
- Cheddar-Stuffed Burgers with Zucchini
- Chicken Cordon Bleu with Cauliflower
- Sesame-Crusted Tuna with Green Beans
- Rosemary Roasted Pork with Cauliflower
- Chicken Tikka with Cauliflower Rice
- Grilled Salmon and Zucchini with Mango Sauce
- Slow-Cooker Pot Roast with Green Beans
- Beef and Broccoli Stir-Fry
- Parmesan-Crusted Halibut with Asparagus
- Hearty Beef and Bacon Casserole
- Sesame Wings with Cauliflower
- Fried Coconut Shrimp with Asparagus
- Coconut Chicken Curry with Cauliflower Rice
- Spicy Chicken Enchilada Casserole
- White Cheddar Broccoli Chicken Casserole
- Sausage Stuffed Bell Peppers
- Cheddar, Sausage, and Mushroom Casserole
- Cauliflower Crust Meat Lover's Pizza
- Slow Cooker Beef Bourguignon
- Pepper Grilled Ribeye with Asparagus
- Bacon-Wrapped Pork Tenderloin with Cauliflower
- Steak Kebabs with Peppers and Onions
- Seared Lamb Chops with Asparagus
- Lemon Chicken Kebabs with Veggies
- Balsamic Salmon with Green Beans

Fat Bomb, Snack and Dessert Recipes

- Pumpkin Spiced Almonds
- Coco-Macadamia Fat Bombs
- Tzatziki Dip with Cauliflower
- Curry-Roasted Macadamia Nuts
- Sesame Almond Fat Bombs
- Overnight Coconut Chia Pudding
- Chocolate Almond Butter Brownies
- Layered Almond Chocolate Fat Bombs

- Bacon Cheeseburger Bites
- Layered Coco-Chia Fat Bombs
- Cinnamon Quick Bread
- Lemon Meringue Cookies
- Almond Flour Cupcakes
- Coconut Macaroons
- Vanilla Coconut Milk Ice Cream
- Crunchy Ginger Cookies
- Vanilla Coconut Milk Flan
- Peppermint Dark Chocolate Fudge
- Layered Choco-Coconut Bars
- Creamy Queso Dip
- Choco-Pistachio Fat Bombs
- Matcha Coconut Fat Bombs
- Coco-Almond Fat Bomb Bars
- Chocolate-Dipped Pecan Fat Bombs
- Dark Chocolate Pistachio Fat Bombs
- Chocolate-Dipped Coconut Fat Bombs
- Chocolate Sunbutter Fat Bombs
- Cinnamon Mug Cake
- Raspberry Coconut Mousse
- Chocolate Coconut Truffles
- Cinnamon-Spiced Pumpkin Bars
- Chocolate Avocado Pudding
- Classic Guacamole Dip
- Cashew Macadamia Fat Bomb Bars

Breakfast

Breakfast Recipes

<u>Sheet Pan Eggs with Veggies and Parmesan</u>

Servings: 6

Prep Time: 5 minutes

Cook Time: 15 minutes

Ingredients:

- 12 large eggs, whisked
- Salt and pepper
- 1 small red pepper, diced
- 1 small yellow onion, chopped
- 1 cup diced mushrooms
- 1 cup diced zucchini
- 1 cup freshly grated parmesan cheese

Instructions:

1. Preheat the oven to 350°F and grease a rimmed baking sheet with cooking spray.
2. Whisk the eggs in a bowl with salt and pepper until frothy.
3. Stir in the peppers, onions, mushrooms, and zucchini until well combined.
4. Pour the mixture in the baking sheet and spread into an even layer.
5. Sprinkle with parmesan and bake for 12 to 15 minutes until the egg is set.
6. Let cool slightly, then cut into squares to serve.

Nutrition Info: 215 calories, 14g fat, 18.5g protein, 5g carbs, 1g fiber, 4g net carbs

Breakfast Recipes

<u>Kale Avocado Smoothie</u>

Servings: 1

Prep Time: 5 minutes

Cook Time: None

Ingredients:

- 1 cup fresh chopped kale
- ½ cup chopped avocado

- ¾ cup unsweetened almond milk
- ¼ cup full-fat yogurt, plain
- 3 to 4 ice cubes
- 1 tablespoon fresh lemon juice
- Liquid stevia extract, to taste

Instructions:

1. Combine the kale, avocado, and almond milk in a blender.
2. Pulse the ingredients several times.
3. Add the remaining ingredients and blend until smooth.
4. Pour into a large glass and enjoy immediately.

Nutrition Info: 250 calories, 19g fat, 6g protein, 17.5g carbs, 6.5g fiber, 11g net carbs

Breakfast Recipes

Almond Butter Protein Smoothie

Servings: 1

Prep Time: 5 minutes

Cook Time: None

Ingredients:

- 1 cup unsweetened almond milk
- ½ cup full-fat yogurt, plain
- ¼ cup vanilla egg white protein powder
- 1 tablespoon almond butter
- Pinch ground cinnamon
- Liquid stevia extract, to taste

Instructions:

1. Combine the almond milk and yogurt in a blender.
2. Pulse the ingredients several times.
3. Add the remaining ingredients and blend until smooth.
4. Pour into a large glass and enjoy immediately.

Nutrition Info: 315 calories, 16.5g fat, 31.5g protein, 12g carbs, 2.5g fiber, 9.5g net carb

Breakfast Recipes

Beets and Blueberry Smoothie

Servings: 1

Prep Time: 5 minutes

Cook Time: None

Ingredients:

- 1 cup unsweetened coconut milk
- ¼ cup heavy cream
- ¼ cup frozen blueberries
- 1 small beet, peeled and chopped
- 1 teaspoon chia seeds
- Liquid stevia extract, to taste

Instructions:

1. Combine the blueberries, beets, and coconut milk in a blender.
2. Pulse the ingredients several times.
3. Add the remaining ingredients and blend until smooth.
4. Pour into a large glass and enjoy immediately.

Nutrition Info: 215 calories, 17g fat, 2.5g protein, 15g carbs, 5g fiber, 10g net carbs

Breakfast Recipes

Almond Butter Muffins

Servings: 12

Prep Time: 10 minutes

Cook Time: 25 minutes

Ingredients:

- 2 cups almond flour
- 1 cup powdered erythritol
- 2 teaspoons baking powder
- ¼ teaspoon salt
- ¾ cup almond butter, warmed
- ¾ cup unsweetened almond milk
- 4 large eggs

Instructions:

1. Preheat the oven to 350°F and line a muffin pan with paper liners.
2. Whisk the almond flour together with the erythritol, baking powder, and salt in a mixing bowl.
3. In a separate bowl, whisk together the almond milk, almond butter, and eggs.
4. Stir the wet ingredients into the dry until just combined.
5. Spoon the batter into the prepared pan and bake for 22 to 25 minutes until a knife inserted in the center comes out clean.
6. Cool the muffins in the pan for 5 minutes then turn out onto a wire cooling rack.

Nutrition Info: 135 calories, 11g fat, 6g protein, 4g carbs, 2g fiber, 2g net carbs

Breakfast Recipes

<u>Classic Western Omelet</u>

Servings: 1

Prep Time: 5 minutes

Cook Time: 10 minutes

Ingredients:

- 2 teaspoons coconut oil
- 3 large eggs, whisked
- 1 tablespoon heavy cream
- Salt and pepper
- ¼ cup diced green pepper
- ¼ cup diced yellow onion
- ¼ cup diced ham

Instructions:

1. Whisk together the eggs, heavy cream, salt and pepper in a small bowl.
2. Heat 1 teaspoon coconut oil in a small skillet over medium heat.
3. Add the peppers, onions, and ham then sauté for 3 to 4 minutes.
4. Spoon the mixture into a bowl and reheat the skillet with the rest of the oil.
5. Pour in the whisked eggs and cook until the bottom of the egg starts to set.
6. Tilt the pan to spread the egg and cook until almost set.
7. Spoon the veggie and ham mixture over half the omelet and fold it over.
8. Let the omelet cook until the eggs are set then serve hot.

Nutrition Info: 415 calories, 32.5g fat, 25g protein, 6.5g carbs, 1.5g fiber, 5g net carbs

Breakfast Recipes

Cinnamon Protein Pancakes

Servings: 4

Prep Time: 5 minutes

Cook Time: 15 minutes

Ingredients:

- 1 cup canned coconut milk
- ¼ cup coconut oil
- 8 large eggs
- 2 scoops (40g) egg white protein powder
- 1 teaspoon vanilla extract
- ½ teaspoon ground cinnamon
- Pinch ground nutmeg
- Liquid stevia extract, to taste

Instructions:

1. Combine the coconut milk, coconut oil, and eggs in a food processor.
2. Pulse the mixture several times then add the remaining ingredients.
3. Blend until smooth and well combined – adjust sweetness to taste.
4. Heat a nonstick skillet over medium heat.
5. Spoon in the batter, using about ¼ cup per pancake.
6. Cook until bubbles form on the surface of the batter then carefully flip.
7. Let the pancake cook until the underside is browned.
8. Transfer to a plate to keep warm and repeat with the remaining batter.

Nutrition Info: 440 calories, 38g fat, 22g protein, 5.5g carbs, 1.5g fiber, 4g net carbs

Breakfast Recipes

Sheet Pan Eggs with Ham and Pepper Jack

Servings: 6

Prep Time: 5 minutes

Cook Time: 15 minutes

Ingredients:

- 12 large eggs, whisked
- Salt and pepper

- 2 cups diced ham
- 1 cup shredded pepper jack cheese

Instructions:

1. Preheat the oven to 350°F and grease a rimmed baking sheet with cooking spray.
2. Whisk the eggs in a bowl with salt and pepper until frothy.
3. Stir in the ham and cheese until well combined.
4. Pour the mixture in the baking sheet and spread into an even layer.
5. Bake for 12 to 15 minutes until the egg is set.
6. Let cool slightly then cut into squares to serve.

Nutrition Info: 235 calories, 15g fat, 21g protein, 2.5g carbs, 0.5g fiber, 2g net carbs

Breakfast Recipes

Detoxifying Green Smoothie

Servings: 1

Prep Time: 5 minutes

Cook Time: None

Ingredients:

- 1 cup fresh chopped kale
- ½ cup fresh baby spinach
- ¼ cup sliced celery
- 1 cup water
- 3 to 4 ice cubes
- 2 tablespoons fresh lemon juice
- 1 tablespoon fresh lime juice
- 1 tablespoon coconut oil
- Liquid stevia extract, to taste

Instructions:

1. Combine the kale, spinach, and celery in a blender.
2. Pulse the ingredients several times.
3. Add the remaining ingredients and blend until smooth.
4. Pour into a large glass and enjoy immediately.

Nutrition Info: 160 calories, 14g fat, 2.5g protein, 8g carbs, 2g fiber, 6g net carbs

Breakfast Recipes

Nutty Pumpkin Smoothie

Servings: 1

Prep Time: 5 minutes

Cook Time: None

Ingredients:

- 1 cup unsweetened cashew milk
- ½ cup pumpkin puree
- ¼ cup heavy cream
- 1 tablespoon raw almonds
- ¼ teaspoon pumpkin pie spice
- Liquid stevia extract, to taste

Instructions:

1. Combine all of the ingredients in a blender.
2. Pulse the ingredients several times, then blend until smooth.
3. Pour into a large glass and enjoy immediately.

Nutrition Info: 205 calories, 16.5g fat, 3g protein, 13g carbs, 4.5g fiber, 8.5g net carbs

Breakfast Recipes

Tomato Mozzarella Egg Muffins

Servings: 12

Prep Time: 5 minutes

Cook Time: 25 minutes

Ingredients:

- 1 tablespoon butter
- 1 medium tomato, finely diced
- ½ cup diced yellow onion
- 12 large eggs, whisked
- ½ cup canned coconut milk
- ¼ cup sliced green onion
- Salt and pepper
- 1 cup shredded mozzarella cheese

Instructions:

1. Preheat the oven to 350°F and grease a muffin pan with cooking spray.
2. Melt the butter in a medium skillet over medium heat.
3. Add the tomato and onions then cook for 3 to 4 minutes until softened.
4. Divide the mixture among the muffin cups.
5. Whisk together the eggs, coconut milk, green onions, salt, and pepper, then spoon into the muffin cups.
6. Sprinkle with cheese then bake for 20 to 25 minutes until the egg is set.

Nutrition Information: 135 calories, 10.5g fat, 9g protein, 2g carbs, 0.5g fiber, 1.5g net carbs

Breakfast Recipes

Crispy Chai Waffles

Servings: 4

Prep Time: 10 minutes

Cook Time: 20 minutes

Ingredients:

- 4 large eggs, separated into whites and yolks
- 3 tablespoons coconut flour
- 3 tablespoons powdered erythritol
- 1 ¼ teaspoon baking powder
- 1 teaspoon vanilla extract
- ½ teaspoon ground cinnamon
- ¼ teaspoon ground ginger
- Pinch ground cloves
- Pinch ground cardamom
- 3 tablespoons coconut oil, melted
- 3 tablespoons unsweetened almond milk

Instructions:

1. Separate the eggs into two different mixing bowls.
2. Whip the egg whites until stiff peaks form then set aside.
3. Whisk the egg yolks with the coconut flour, erythritol, baking powder, vanilla, cinnamon, cardamom, and cloves in the other bowl.
4. Add the melted coconut oil to the second bowl while whisking then whisk in the almond milk.
5. Gently fold in the egg whites until just combined.
6. Preheat the waffle iron and grease with cooking spray.
7. Spoon about ½ cup of batter into the iron.

8. Cook the waffle according to the manufacturer's instructions.
9. Remove the waffle to a plate and repeat with the remaining batter.

Nutrition Info: 215 calories, 17g fat, 8g protein, 8g carbs, 4g fiber, 4g net carbs

Breakfast Recipes

<u>Broccoli Kale Egg Scramble</u>

Servings: 1

Prep Time: 5 minutes

Cook Time: 10 minutes

Ingredients:

- 2 large eggs, whisked
- 1 tablespoon heavy cream
- Salt and pepper
- 1 teaspoon coconut oil
- 1 cup fresh chopped kale
- ¼ cup frozen broccoli florets, thawed
- 2 tablespoons grated parmesan cheese

Instructions:

1. Whisk the eggs together with the heavy cream, salt, and pepper in a bowl.
2. Heat 1 teaspoon coconut oil in a medium skillet over medium heat.
3. Stir in the kale and broccoli then cook until the kale is wilted, about 1 to 2 minutes.
4. Pour in the eggs and cook, stirring occasionally, until just set.
5. Stir in the parmesan cheese and serve hot.

Nutrition Info: 315 calories, 23g fat, 19.5g protein, 10g carbs, 1.5g fiber, 8.5g net carbs

Breakfast Recipes

<u>Creamy Chocolate Protein Smoothie</u>

Servings: 1

Prep Time: 5 minutes

Cook Time: None

Ingredients:

- 1 cup unsweetened almond milk
- ½ cup full-fat yogurt, plain

- ¼ cup chocolate egg white protein powder
- 1 tablespoon coconut oil
- 1 tablespoon unsweetened cocoa powder
- Liquid stevia extract, to taste

Instructions:

1. Combine the almond milk, yogurt, and protein powder in a blender.
2. Pulse the ingredients several times then add the rest and blend until smooth.
3. Pour into a large glass and enjoy immediately.

Nutrition Info: 345 calories, 22g fat, 29g protein, 12g carbs, 3g fiber, 9g net carbs

Breakfast Recipes

<u>Three Cheese Egg Muffins</u>

Servings: 12

Prep Time: 5 minutes

Cook Time: 25 minutes

Ingredients:

- 1 tablespoon butter
- ½ cup diced yellow onion
- 12 large eggs, whisked
- ½ cup canned coconut milk
- ¼ cup sliced green onion
- Salt and pepper
- ½ cup shredded cheddar cheese
- ½ cup shredded Swiss cheese
- ¼ cup grated parmesan cheese

Instructions:

1. Preheat the oven to 350°F and grease a muffin pan with cooking spray.
2. Melt the butter in a medium skillet over medium heat.
3. Add the onions then cook for 3 to 4 minutes until softened.
4. Divide the mixture among the muffin cups.
5. Whisk together the eggs, coconut milk, green onions, salt, and pepper, then spoon into the muffin cups.
6. Combine the three cheeses in a bowl and sprinkle over the egg muffins.
7. Bake for 20 to 25 minutes until the egg is set.

Nutrition Information: 150 calories, 11.5g fat, 10g protein, 2g carbs, 0.5g fiber, 1.5g net carbs

Breakfast Recipes

<u>Strawberry Rhubarb Pie Smoothie</u>

Servings: 1

Prep Time: 5 minutes

Cook Time: None

Ingredients:

- 1 small stalk rhubarb, sliced
- ¼ cup frozen sliced strawberries
- ¾ cup unsweetened cashew milk
- ½ cup full-fat yogurt, plain
- 1 ounce raw almonds
- ½ teaspoon vanilla extract
- Liquid stevia extract, to taste

Instructions:

1. Combine the rhubarb, strawberries, and almond milk in a blender.
2. Pulse the ingredients several times.
3. Add the remaining ingredients and blend until smooth.
4. Pour into a large glass and enjoy immediately.

Nutrition Info: 285 calories, 20g fat, 11g protein, 17.5g carbs, 5g fiber, 12.5g net carbs

Breakfast Recipes

<u>Vanilla Chai Smoothie</u>

Servings: 1

Prep Time: 5 minutes

Cook Time: None

Ingredients:

- 1 cup unsweetened almond milk
- ½ cup full-fat yogurt, plain
- 1 teaspoon vanilla extract

- ¼ teaspoon ground cinnamon
- ¼ teaspoon ground ginger
- Pinch ground cloves
- Pinch ground cardamom
- Liquid stevia extract, to taste

Instructions:

1. Combine all of the ingredients in a blender.
2. Pulse the ingredients several times then blend smooth.
3. Pour into a large glass and enjoy immediately.

Nutrition Info: 115 calories, 7.5g fat, 5g protein, 7.5g carbs, 1g fiber, 6.5g net carbs

Breakfast Recipes

Cinnamon Almond Porridge

Servings: 1

Prep Time: 5 minutes

Cook Time: 5 minutes

Ingredients:

- 1 tablespoon butter
- 1 tablespoon coconut flour
- 1 large egg, whisked
- ⅛ teaspoon ground cinnamon
- Pinch salt
- ¼ cup canned coconut milk
- 1 tablespoon almond butter

Instructions:

1. Melt the butter in a small saucepan over low heat.
2. Whisk in the coconut flour, egg, cinnamon, and salt.
3. Add the coconut milk while whisking and stir in the almond butter until smooth.
4. Simmer on low heat, stirring often, until heated through.
5. Spoon into a bowl and serve.

Nutrition Info: 470 calories, 42g fat, 13g protein, 15g carbs, 8g fiber, 7g net carbs

Breakfast Recipes

Bacon, Mushroom, and Swiss Omelet

Servings: 1

Prep Time: 5 minutes

Cook Time: 10 minutes

Ingredients:

- 3 large eggs, whisked
- 1 tablespoon heavy cream
- Salt and pepper
- 2 slices uncooked bacon, chopped
- ¼ cup diced mushrooms
- ¼ cup shredded Swiss cheese

Instructions:

1. Whisk together the eggs, heavy cream, salt, and pepper in a small bowl.
2. Cook the bacon in a small skillet over medium-high heat.
3. When the bacon is crisp, spoon it into a bowl.
4. Reheat the skillet over medium heat, then add the mushrooms.
5. Cook the mushrooms until browned, then spoon into the bowl with the bacon.
6. Reheat the skillet with the rest of the oil.
7. Pour in the whisked eggs and cook until the bottom of the egg starts to set.
8. Tilt the pan to spread the egg and cook until almost set.
9. Spoon the bacon and mushroom mixture over half the omelet then sprinkle with cheese and fold it over.
10. Let the omelet cook until the eggs are set, then serve hot.

Nutrition Info: 475 calories, 36g fat, 34g protein, 4g carbs, 0.5g fiber, 3.5g net carbs

Breakfast Recipes

Maple Cranberry Muffins

Servings: 12

Prep Time: 10 minutes

Cook Time: 20 minutes

Ingredients:

- ¾ cups almond flour

- ¼ cup ground flaxseed
- ¼ cup powdered erythritol
- 1 teaspoon baking powder
- ⅛ teaspoon salt
- ⅓ cup canned coconut milk
- ¼ cup coconut oil, melted
- 3 large eggs
- ½ cup fresh cranberries
- 1 teaspoon maple extract

Instructions:

1. Preheat the oven to 350°F and line a muffin pan with paper liners.
2. Whisk the almond flour together with the ground flaxseed, erythritol, baking powder, and salt in a mixing bowl.
3. In a separate bowl, whisk together the coconut milk, coconut oil, eggs, and maple extract.
4. Stir the wet ingredients into the dry until just combined, then fold in the cranberries.
5. Spoon the batter into the prepared pan and bake for 18 to 20 minutes until a knife inserted in the center comes out clean.
6. Cool the muffins in the pan for 5 minutes, then turn out onto a wire cooling rack.

Nutrition Info: 125 calories, 11.5g fat, 3.5g protein, 3g carbs, 1.5g fiber, 1.5g net carbs

Breakfast Recipes

Coco-Cashew Macadamia Muffins

Servings: 12

Prep Time: 10 minutes

Cook Time: 25 minutes

Ingredients:

- 1 ¾ cups almond flour
- 1 cup powdered erythritol
- ¼ cup unsweetened cocoa powder
- 2 teaspoons baking powder
- ¼ teaspoon salt
- ¾ cup cashew butter, melted
- ¾ cup unsweetened almond milk
- 4 large eggs
- ¼ cup chopped macadamia nuts

Instructions:

1. Preheat the oven to 350°F and line a muffin pan with paper liners.
2. Whisk the almond flour together with the erythritol, cocoa powder, baking powder, and salt in a mixing bowl.
3. In a separate bowl, whisk together the almond milk, cashew butter, and eggs.
4. Stir the wet ingredients into the dry until just combined then fold in the nuts.
5. Spoon the batter into the prepared pan and bake for 22 to 25 minutes until a knife inserted in the center comes out clean.
6. Cool the muffins in the pan for 5 minutes then turn out onto a wire cooling rack.

Nutrition Info: 230 calories, 20g fat, 9g protein, 9g carbs, 2.5g fiber, 6.5g net carbs

Breakfast Recipes

Chocolate Protein Pancakes

Servings: 4

Prep Time: 5 minutes

Cook Time: 15 minutes

Ingredients:

- 1 cup canned coconut milk
- ¼ cup coconut oil
- 8 large eggs
- 2 scoops (40g) egg white protein powder
- ¼ cup unsweetened cocoa powder
- 1 teaspoon vanilla extract
- Liquid stevia extract, to taste

Instructions:

1. Combine the coconut milk, coconut oil, and eggs in a food processor.
2. Pulse the mixture several times then add the remaining ingredients.
3. Blend until smooth and well combined – adjust sweetness to taste.
4. Heat a nonstick skillet over medium heat.
5. Spoon in the batter, using about ¼ cup per pancake.
6. Cook until bubbles form on the surface of the batter, then carefully flip.
7. Let the pancake cook until the underside is browned.
8. Transfer to a plate to keep warm and repeat with the remaining batter.

Nutrition Info: 455 calories, 38.5g fat, 23g protein, 8g carbs, 3g fiber, 5g net carbs

Breakfast Recipes

Ham, Cheddar, and Chive Omelet

Servings: 1

Prep Time: 5 minutes

Cook Time: 10 minutes

Ingredients:

- 1 teaspoon coconut oil
- 3 large eggs, whisked
- 1 tablespoon heavy cream
- 1 tablespoon chopped chives
- Salt and pepper
- ¼ cup shredded cheddar cheese
- ¼ cup diced ham

Instructions:

1. Whisk together the eggs, heavy cream, chives, salt, and pepper in a small bowl.
2. Heat the coconut oil in a small skillet over medium heat.
3. Pour in the whisked eggs and cook until the bottom of the egg starts to set.
4. Tilt the pan to spread the egg and cook until almost set.
5. Sprinkle the ham and cheddar cheese over half the omelet and fold it over.
6. Let the omelet cook until the eggs are set, then serve hot.

Nutrition Info: 515 calories, 42g fat, 32g protein, 3.5g carbs, 0.5g fiber, 3g net carbs

Breakfast Recipes

Spinach Parmesan Egg Scramble

Servings: 1

Prep Time: 5 minutes

Cook Time: 10 minutes

Ingredients:

- 2 large eggs, whisked
- 1 tablespoon heavy cream
- Salt and pepper
- 1 teaspoon coconut oil
- 2 cups fresh baby spinach

- 2 tablespoons grated parmesan cheese

Instructions:

1. Whisk the eggs together with the heavy cream, salt, and pepper in a bowl.
2. Heat the coconut oil in a medium skillet over medium heat.
3. Stir in the spinach and cook until wilted, about 1 to 2 minutes.
4. Pour in the eggs and cook, stirring occasionally, until just set – about 1 to 2 minutes.
5. Stir in the parmesan and serve hot.

Nutrition Info: 290 calories, 23g fat, 18.5g protein, 3.5g carbs, 1.5g fiber, 2g net carbs

Breakfast Recipes

Cinnamon Roll Waffles

Servings: 2

Prep Time: 10 minutes

Cook Time: 20 minutes

Ingredients:

- 4 large eggs, separated into whites and yolks
- 3 tablespoons coconut flour
- 3 tablespoons powdered erythritol
- 1 ¼ teaspoon baking powder
- 1 teaspoon vanilla extract
- ½ teaspoon ground cinnamon
- Pinch ground nutmeg
- ½ cup heavy cream

Instructions:

1. Separate the eggs into two different mixing bowls.
2. Whip the egg whites until stiff peaks form then set aside.
3. Whisk the egg yolks with the coconut flour, erythritol, baking powder, vanilla, cinnamon, and nutmeg in the other bowl.
4. Add the heavy cream, whisking until just combined, then gently fold in the egg whites.
5. Preheat the waffle iron and grease with cooking spray.
6. Spoon about ½ cup of batter into the iron.
7. Cook the waffle according to the manufacturer's instructions.
8. Remove the waffle to a plate and repeat with the remaining batter.

Nutrition Info: 350 calories, 24g fat, 16g protein, 16g carbs, 8g fiber, 8g net carbs

Breakfast Recipes

Bacon Swiss Waffles

Servings: 4

Prep Time: 10 minutes

Cook Time: 20 minutes

Ingredients:

- 6 slices uncooked bacon
- 4 large eggs, separated into whites and yolks
- 3 tablespoons coconut flour
- 1 ¼ teaspoon baking powder
- Salt and pepper
- 3 tablespoons unsweetened almond milk
- ½ cup shredded Swiss cheese
- ¼ cup sour cream

Instructions:

1. Cook the bacon in a skillet until crisp then coarsely chop into a bowl.
2. Spoon out 3 tablespoons of the bacon grease and set it aside.
3. Separate the eggs into two different mixing bowls.
4. Whip the egg whites until stiff peaks form then set aside.
5. Whisk the egg yolks with the coconut flour, erythritol, baking powder, salt, and pepper in the other bowl.
6. Add the almond milk and bacon grease to the second bowl while whisking then gently fold in the egg whites until just combined.
7. Stir in the shredded Swiss cheese and half the chopped bacon.
8. Preheat the waffle iron and grease with cooking spray.
9. Spoon a heaping ½ cup of batter into the iron.
10. Cook the waffle according to the manufacturer's instructions.
11. Remove the waffle to a plate and repeat with the remaining batter.
12. Serve the waffles topped with sour cream and chopped bacon.

Nutrition Info: 250 calories, 16.5g fat, 17g protein, 8g carbs, 4g fiber, 4g net carbs

Breakfast Recipes

Meaty Breakfast Omelet

Servings: 1

Prep Time: 5 minutes

Cook Time: 10 minutes

Ingredients:

- 3 large eggs, whisked
- 1 tablespoon heavy cream
- Salt and pepper
- 1 slice uncooked bacon, chopped
- 1 ounce breakfast sausage, crumbled
- ¼ cup diced ham

Instructions:

1. Whisk together the eggs, heavy cream, salt, and pepper in a small bowl.
2. Cook the bacon in a small skillet over medium-high heat.
3. When the bacon is crisp, spoon it off into a bowl.
4. Cook the sausage in the skillet until browned, then add to the bowl with the bacon.
5. Reheat the skillet with the grease from the bacon and sausage.
6. Pour in the whisked eggs and cook until the bottom of the egg starts to set.
7. Tilt the pan to spread the egg and cook until almost set.
8. Sprinkle the bacon, sausage, and ham over half the omelet and fold it over.
9. Let the omelet cook until the eggs are set, then serve hot.

Nutrition Info: 470 calories, 35.5g fat, 34g protein, 3g carbs, 0.5g fiber, 2.5g net carbs

Breakfast Recipes

Lemon Flaxseed Muffins

Servings: 12

Prep Time: 10 minutes

Cook Time: 20 minutes

Ingredients:

- ¾ cups almond flour
- ¼ cup ground flaxseed
- ¼ cup powdered erythritol
- 1 teaspoon baking powder
- ⅛ teaspoon salt
- ¼ cup canned coconut milk
- ¼ cup coconut oil, melted
- ¼ cup fresh lemon juice
- 3 large eggs
- 2 tablespoons grated lemon peel

Instructions:

1. Preheat the oven to 350°F and line a muffin pan with paper liners.
2. Whisk the almond flour together with the ground flaxseed, erythritol, baking powder, and salt in a mixing bowl.
3. In a separate bowl, whisk together the coconut milk, coconut oil, lemon juice, and eggs.
4. Stir the wet ingredients into the dry until just combined.
5. Fold in the grated lemon peel.
6. Spoon the batter into the prepared pan and bake for 18 to 20 minutes until a knife inserted in the center comes out clean.
7. Cool the muffins in the pan for 5 minutes, then turn out onto a wire cooling rack.

Nutrition Info: 120 calories, 11g fat, 3.5g protein, 3g carbs, 1.5g fiber, 1.5g net carbs

Breakfast Recipes

<u>Pumpkin Spice Waffles</u>

Servings: 2

Prep Time: 10 minutes

Cook Time: 20 minutes

Ingredients:

- 4 large eggs, separated into whites and yolks
- 3 tablespoons coconut flour
- 3 tablespoons powdered erythritol
- 1 ¼ teaspoon baking powder
- 1 teaspoon vanilla extract
- ½ teaspoon ground cinnamon
- ¼ teaspoon ground nutmeg
- Pinch ground cloves
- ½ cup pumpkin puree

Instructions:

1. Separate the eggs into two different mixing bowls.
2. Whip the egg whites until stiff peaks form then set aside.
3. Whisk the egg yolks with the coconut flour, erythritol, baking powder, vanilla, cinnamon, nutmeg, and cloves in the other bowl.
4. Add the pumpkin puree, whisking until combined, then gently fold in the egg whites.
5. Preheat the waffle iron and grease with cooking spray.
6. Spoon about ½ cup of batter into the iron.
7. Cook the waffle according to the manufacturer's instructions.
8. Remove the waffle to a plate and repeat with the remaining batter.

Nutrition Info: 265 calories, 13.5g fat, 16g protein, 20g carbs, 10g fiber, 10g net carbs

Lunch

Lunch Recipes

Cucumber Avocado Salad with Bacon

Servings: 2

Prep Time: 10 minutes

Cook Time: None

Ingredients:

- 2 cups fresh baby spinach, chopped
- ½ English cucumber, sliced thin
- 1 small avocado, pitted and chopped
- 1 ½ tablespoons olive oil
- 1 ½ tablespoons lemon juice
- Salt and pepper
- 2 slices cooked bacon, chopped

Instructions:

1. Combine the spinach, cucumber, and avocado in a salad bowl.
2. Toss with the olive oil, lemon juice, salt and pepper.
3. Top with chopped bacon to serve.

Nutrition Info: 365 calories, 24.5g fat, 7g protein, 13g carbs, 8g fiber, 5g net carbs

Lunch Recipes

Bacon Cheeseburger Soup

Servings: 4

Prep Time: 10 minutes

Cook Time: 15 minutes

Ingredients:

- 4 slices uncooked bacon
- 8 ounces ground beef (80% lean)
- 1 medium yellow onion, chopped

- 1 clove garlic, minced
- 3 cups beef broth
- 2 tablespoons tomato paste
- 2 teaspoons Dijon mustard
- Salt and pepper
- 1 cup shredded lettuce
- ½ cup shredded cheddar cheese

Instructions:

1. Cook the bacon in a saucepan until crisp then drain on paper towels and chop.
2. Reheat the bacon fat in the saucepan and add the beef.
3. Cook until the beef is browned, then drain away half the fat.
4. Reheat the saucepan and add the onion and garlic – cook for 6 minutes.
5. Stir in the broth, tomato paste, and mustard then season with salt and pepper.
6. Add the beef and simmer on medium-low for 15 minutes, covered.
7. Spoon into bowls and top with shredded lettuce, cheddar cheese and bacon.

Nutrition Info: 315 calories, 20g fat, 27g protein, 6g carbs, 1g fiber, 5g net carbs

Lunch Recipes

Ham and Provolone Sandwich

Servings: 1

Prep Time: 30 minutes

Cook Time: 5 minutes

Ingredients:

- 1 large egg, separated
- Pinch cream of tartar
- Pinch salt
- 1 ounce cream cheese, softened
- ¼ cup shredded provolone cheese
- 3 ounces sliced ham

Instructions:

1. For the bread, preheat the oven to 300°F and line a baking sheet with parchment.
2. Beat the egg whites with the cream of tartar and salt until soft peaks form.
3. Whisk the cream cheese and egg yolk until smooth and pale yellow.
4. Fold in the egg whites a little at a time until smooth and well combined.
5. Spoon the batter onto the baking sheet into two even circles.
6. Bake for 25 minutes until firm and lightly browned.

7. Spread the butter on one side of each bread circle then place one in a preheated skillet over medium heat.
8. Sprinkle with cheese and add the sliced ham then top with the other bread circle, butter-side-up.
9. Cook the sandwich for a minute or two then carefully flip it over.
10. Let it cook until the cheese is melted then serve.

Nutrition Info: 425 calories, 31g fat, 31g protein, 5g carbs, 1g fiber, 4g net carbs

Lunch Recipes

<u>Baked Chicken Nuggets</u>

Servings: 4

Prep Time: 10 minutes

Cook Time: 20 minutes

Ingredients:

- ¼ cup almond flour
- 1 teaspoon chili powder
- ½ teaspoon paprika
- 2 pounds boneless chicken thighs, cut into 2-inch chunks
- Salt and pepper
- 2 large eggs, whisked well

Instructions:

1. Preheat the oven to 400°F and line a baking sheet with parchment.
2. Stir together the almond flour, chili powder, and paprika in a shallow dish.
3. Season the chicken with salt and pepper, then dip in the beaten eggs.
4. Dredge the chicken pieces in the almond flour mixture, then arrange on the baking sheet.
5. Bake for 20 minutes until browned and crisp. Serve hot.

Nutrition Info: 400 calories, 26g fat, 43g protein, 2g carbs, 1g fiber, 1g net carbs

Lunch Recipes

<u>Taco Salad with Creamy Dressing</u>

Servings: 2

Prep Time: 10 minutes

Cook Time: 10 minutes

Ingredients:

- 6 ounces ground beef (80% lean)
- Salt and pepper
- 1 tablespoon ground cumin
- 1 tablespoon chili powder
- 4 cups fresh chopped lettuce
- ½ cup diced tomatoes
- ¼ cup diced red onion
- ¼ cup shredded cheddar cheese
- 3 tablespoons mayonnaise
- 1 teaspoon apple cider vinegar
- Pinch paprika

Instructions:

1. Cook the ground beef in a skillet over medium-high heat until browned.
2. Drain half the fat, then season with salt and pepper and stir in the taco seasoning.
3. Simmer for 5 minutes, then remove from heat.
4. Divide the lettuce between two salad bowls, then top with ground beef.
5. Add the diced tomatoes, red onion, and cheddar cheese.
6. Whisk together the remaining ingredients, then drizzle over the salads to serve.

Nutrition Info: 470 calories, 36g fat, 28g protein, 7.5g carbs, 1.5g fiber, 6g net carbs

Lunch Recipes

Egg Salad Over Lettuce

Servings: 2

Prep Time: 10 minutes

Cook Time: None

Ingredients:

- 3 large hardboiled eggs, cooled
- 1 small stalk celery, diced
- 3 tablespoons mayonnaise
- 1 tablespoon fresh chopped parsley
- 1 teaspoon fresh lemon juice
- Salt and pepper
- 4 cups fresh chopped lettuce

Instructions:

1. Peel and dice the eggs into a mixing bowl.
2. Stir in the celery, mayonnaise, parsley, lemon juice, salt and pepper.
3. Serve spooned over fresh chopped lettuce.

Nutrition Info: 260 calories, 23g fat, 10g protein, 4g carbs, 1g fiber, 3g net carbs

Lunch Recipes

Egg Drop Soup

Servings: 4

Prep Time: 5 minutes

Cook Time: 10 minutes

Ingredients:

- 5 cups chicken broth
- 4 chicken bouillon cubes
- 1 ½ tablespoons chili garlic paste
- 6 large eggs, whisked
- ½ green onion, sliced

Instructions:

1. Crush the bouillon cubes and stir into the broth in a saucepan.
2. Bring it to a boil, then stir in the chili garlic paste.
3. Cook until steaming, then remove from heat.
4. While whisking, drizzle in the beaten eggs.
5. Let sit for 2 minutes then serve with sliced green onion.

Nutrition Info: 165 calories, 9.5g fat, 16g protein, 2.5g carbs, 0g fiber, 2.5g carbs

Lunch Recipes

Bacon, Lettuce, Tomato, Avocado Sandwich

Servings: 1

Prep Time: 30 minutes

Cook Time: None

Ingredients:

- 1 large egg, separated
- Pinch cream of tartar
- Pinch salt

- 1 ounce cream cheese, softened
- 2 slices uncooked bacon
- ¼ cup sliced avocado
- ¼ cup shredded lettuce
- 1 slice tomato

Instructions:

1. For the bread, preheat the oven to 300°F and line a baking sheet with parchment.
2. Beat the egg whites with the cream of tartar and salt until soft peaks form.
3. Whisk the cream cheese and egg yolk until smooth and pale yellow.
4. Fold in the egg whites a little at a time until smooth and well combined.
5. Spoon the batter onto the baking sheet into two even circles.
6. Bake for 25 minutes until firm and lightly browned.
7. Cook the bacon in a skillet until crisp, then drain on a paper towel.
8. Assemble the sandwich with the bacon, avocado, lettuce, and tomato.

Nutrition Info: 355 calories, 30g fat, 16.5g protein, 5.5g carbs, 2.5g fiber, 3g net carbs

Lunch Recipes

Fried Salmon Cakes

Servings: 2

Prep Time: 15 minutes

Cook Time: 10 minutes

Ingredients:

- 1 tablespoon butter
- 1 cup riced cauliflower
- Salt and pepper
- 8 ounces boneless salmon fillet
- ¼ cup almond flour
- 2 tablespoons coconut flour
- 1 large egg
- 2 tablespoons minced red onion
- 1 tablespoon fresh chopped parsley
- 2 tablespoons coconut oil

Instructions:

1. Melt the butter in a skillet over medium heat, then cook the cauliflower for 5 minutes until tender – season with salt and pepper.
2. Spoon the cauliflower into a bowl and reheat the skillet.

3. Add the salmon and season with salt and pepper.
4. Cook the salmon until just opaque, then remove and flake the fish into a bowl.
5. Stir in the cauliflower along with the almond flour, coconut flour, egg, red onion, and parsley.
6. Shape into 6 patties then fry in coconut oil until both sides are browned.

Nutrition Info: 505 calories, 37.5g fat, 31g protein, 14.5g carbs, 8g fiber, 6.5g net carbs

Lunch Recipes

<u>Spring Salad with Shaved Parmesan</u>

Servings: 2

Prep Time: 15 minutes

Cook Time: None

Ingredients:

- 3 slices uncooked bacon
- 2 tablespoons red wine vinegar
- 1 tablespoon Dijon mustard
- Salt and pepper
- Liquid stevia extract, to taste
- 4 ounces mixed spring greens
- ½ small red onion, sliced thinly
- ⅓ cup roasted pine nuts
- ¼ cup shaved parmesan

Instructions:

1. Cook the bacon in a skillet until crisp then remove to paper towels.
2. Reserve ¼ cup of bacon fat in the skillet, discarding the rest, then chop the bacon.
3. Whisk the red wine vinegar and mustard into the bacon fat in the skillet.
4. Season with salt and pepper, then sweeten with stevia to taste and let cool slightly.
5. Combine the spring greens, red onion, pine nuts, and parmesan in a salad bowl.
6. Toss with the dressing, then top with chopped bacon to serve.

Nutrition Info: 295 calories, 25g fat, 14.5g protein, 6.5g carbs, 3g fiber, 3.5g net carbs

Lunch Recipes

<u>Sesame Chicken Avocado Salad</u>

Servings: 2

Prep Time: 10 minutes

Cook Time: None

Ingredients:

- 1 tablespoon sesame oil
- 8 ounces boneless chicken thighs, chopped
- Salt and pepper
- 4 cups fresh spring greens
- 1 cup sliced avocado
- 2 tablespoons olive oil
- 2 tablespoons rice wine vinegar
- 1 tablespoon sesame seeds

Instructions:

1. Heat the sesame oil in a skillet over medium-high heat.
2. Season the chicken with salt and pepper, then add to the skillet.
3. Cook the chicken until browned and cooked through, stirring often.
4. Remove the chicken from the heat and cool slightly.
5. Divide the spring greens onto two salad plates and top with avocado.
6. Drizzle the salads with olive oil and rice wine vinegar.
7. Top with cooked chicken and sprinkle with sesame seeds to serve.

Nutrition Info: 540 calories, 47.5g fat, 23g protein, 10.5g carbs, 8g fiber, 2.5g net carbs

Lunch Recipes

Spinach Cauliflower Soup

Servings: 4

Prep Time: 5 minutes

Cook Time: 15 minutes

Ingredients:

- 1 tablespoon coconut oil
- 1 small yellow onion, chopped
- 2 cloves garlic, minced
- 2 cups chopped cauliflower
- 8 ounces fresh baby spinach, chopped
- 3 cups vegetable broth
- ½ cup canned coconut milk
- Salt and pepper

Instructions:

1. Heat the oil in a saucepan over medium-high heat – add the onion and garlic.
2. Sauté for 4 to 5 minutes until browned, then stir in the cauliflower.
3. Cook for 5 minutes until browned, then stir in the spinach.
4. Let it cook for 2 minutes until wilted, then stir in the broth and bring to boil.
5. Remove from heat and puree the soup with an immersion blender.
6. Stir in the coconut milk and season with salt and pepper to taste. Serve hot.

Nutrition Info: 165 calories, 12g fat, 7g protein, 9g carbs, 3.5g fiber, 5.5g net carbs

Lunch Recipes

Cheesy Buffalo Chicken Sandwich

Servings: 1

Prep Time: 30 minutes

Cook Time: None

Ingredients:

- 1 large egg, separated into white and yolk
- Pinch cream of tartar
- Pinch salt
- 1 ounce cream cheese, softened
- 1 cup cooked chicken breast, shredded
- 2 tablespoons hot sauce
- 1 slice Swiss cheese

Instructions:

1. For the bread, preheat the oven to 300°F and line a baking sheet with parchment.
2. Beat the egg whites with the cream of tartar and salt until soft peaks form.
3. Whisk the cream cheese and egg yolk until smooth and pale yellow.
4. Fold in the egg whites a little at a time until smooth and well combined.
5. Spoon the batter onto the baking sheet into two even circles.
6. Bake for 25 minutes until firm and lightly browned.
7. Shred the chicken into a bowl and toss with the hot sauce.
8. Spoon the chicken onto one of the bread circles and top with cheese.
9. Top with the other bread circle and enjoy.

Nutrition Info: 555 calories, 33.5g fat, 58g protein, 3.5g carbs, 0g fiber, 3.5g net carbs

Lunch Recipes

Coconut Chicken Tenders

Servings: 4

Prep Time: 10 minutes

Cook Time: 30 minutes

Ingredients:

- ¼ cup almond flour
- 2 tablespoons shredded unsweetened coconut
- ½ teaspoon garlic powder
- 2 pounds boneless chicken tenders
- Salt and pepper
- 2 large eggs, whisked well

Instructions:

1. Preheat the oven to 400°F and line a baking sheet with parchment.
2. Stir together the almond flour, coconut, and garlic powder in a shallow dish.
3. Season the chicken with salt and pepper, then dip into the beaten eggs.
4. Dredge the chicken tenders in the almond flour mixture, then arrange on the baking sheet.
5. Bake for 25 to 30 minutes until browned and cooked through. Serve hot.

Nutrition Info: 325 calories, 9.5g fat, 56.5g protein, 2g carbs, 1g fiber, 1g net carbs

Lunch Recipes

Avocado Spinach Salad with Almonds

Servings: 2

Prep Time: 10 minutes

Cook Time: None

Ingredients:

- 4 cups fresh baby spinach
- 2 tablespoons olive oil
- 1 ½ tablespoons balsamic vinegar
- ½ tablespoon Dijon mustard
- Salt and pepper
- 1 medium avocado, sliced thinly

- ¼ cup sliced almonds, toasted

Instructions:

1. Toss the spinach with the olive oil, balsamic vinegar, Dijon mustard, salt and pepper.
2. Divide the spinach between two salad plates.
3. Top the salads with sliced avocado and toasted almonds to serve.

Nutrition Info: 415 calories, 40g fat, 6.5g protein, 14g carbs, 10g fiber, 4g net carbs

Lunch Recipes

Easy Chopped Salad

Servings: 2

Prep Time: 15 minutes

Cook Time: None

Ingredients:

- 4 cups fresh chopped lettuce
- 1 small avocado, pitted and chopped
- ½ cup cherry tomatoes, halved
- ¼ cup diced cucumber
- 2 hardboiled eggs, peeled and sliced
- 1 cup diced ham
- ½ cup shredded cheddar cheese

Instructions:

1. Divide the lettuce between two salad plates or bowls.
2. Top the salads with diced avocado, tomato, and celery.
3. Add the sliced egg, diced ham, and shredded cheese.
4. Serve the salads with your favorite keto-friendly dressing.

Nutrition Info: 520 calories, 39.5g fat, 27g protein, 17.5g carbs, 9g fiber, 8.5g net carbs

Lunch Recipes

Cauliflower Leek Soup with Pancetta

Servings: 4

Prep Time: 15 minutes

Cook Time: 1 hour

Ingredients:

- 4 cups chicken broth
- ½ medium head cauliflower, chopped
- 1 cup sliced leeks
- ½ cup heavy cream
- Salt and pepper
- 2 ounces diced pancetta

Instructions:

1. Combine the broth and cauliflower in a saucepan over medium-high heat.
2. Bring the chicken broth to a boil then add the sliced leeks.
3. Boil on medium heat, covered, for 1 hour until the cauliflower is tender.
4. Remove from heat and puree the soup with an immersion blender.
5. Stir in the cream, then season with salt and pepper.
6. Fry the chopped pancetta in a skillet over medium-high heat until crisp.
7. Spoon the soup into bowls and sprinkle with pancetta to serve.

Nutrition Info: 200 calories, 13g fat, 12g protein, 8.5g carbs, 2g fiber, 6.5g net carbs

Lunch Recipes

Three Meat and Cheese Sandwich

Servings: 1

Prep Time: 30 minutes

Cook Time: 5 minutes

Ingredients:

- 1 large egg, separated
- Pinch cream of tartar
- Pinch salt
- 1 ounce cream cheese, softened
- 1 ounce sliced ham
- 1 ounce sliced hard salami
- 1 ounce sliced turkey
- 2 slices cheddar cheese

Instructions:

1. For the bread, preheat the oven to 300°F and line a baking sheet with parchment.
2. Beat the egg whites with the cream of tartar and salt until soft peaks form.
3. Whisk the cream cheese and egg yolk until smooth and pale yellow.
4. Fold in the egg whites a little at a time until smooth and well combined.
5. Spoon the batter onto the baking sheet into two even circles.

6. Bake for 25 minutes until firm and lightly browned.
7. To complete the sandwich, layer the sliced meats and cheeses between the two bread circles.
8. Grease a skillet with cooking spray and heat over medium heat.
9. Add the sandwich and cook until browned underneath, then flip and cook until the cheese is just melted.

Nutrition Info: 610 calories, 48g fat, 40g protein, 3g carbs, 0.5g fiber, 2.5g net carbs

Lunch Recipes

Beef and Pepper Kebabs

Servings: 2

Prep Time: 30 minutes

Cook Time: 10 minutes

Ingredients:

- 2 tablespoons olive oil
- 1 ½ tablespoons balsamic vinegar
- 2 teaspoons Dijon mustard
- Salt and pepper
- 8 ounces beef sirloin, cut into 2-inch pieces
- 1 small red pepper, cut into chunks
- 1 small green pepper, cut into chunks

Instructions:

1. Whisk together the olive oil, balsamic vinegar, and mustard in a shallow dish.
2. Season the steak with salt and pepper, then toss in the marinade.
3. Let marinate for 30 minutes, then slide onto skewers with the peppers.
4. Preheat a grill pan to high heat and grease with cooking spray.
5. Cook the kebabs for 2 to 3 minutes on each side until the beef is done.

Nutrition Info: 365 calories, 21.5g fat, 35.5g protein, 6.5g carbs, 1.5g fiber, 5g net carbs

Lunch Recipes

Simple Tuna Salad on Lettuce

Servings: 2

Prep Time: 10 minutes

Cook Time: None

Ingredients:

- ¼ cup mayonnaise
- 1 tablespoon fresh lemon juice
- 1 tablespoon pickle relish
- 2 (6-ounce) cans tuna in oil, drained and flaked
- ½ cup cherry tomatoes, halved
- ¼ cup diced cucumber
- Salt and pepper
- 4 cups chopped romaine lettuce

Instructions:

1. Whisk together the mayonnaise, lemon juice, and relish in a bowl.
2. Toss in the flaked tuna, tomatoes, and cucumber – season with salt and pepper.
3. Spoon over chopped lettuce to serve.

Nutrition Info: 550 calories, 35g fat, 48g protein, 8.5g carbs, 1.5g fiber, 7g net carbs

Lunch Recipes

Ham, Egg, and Cheese Sandwich

Servings: 1

Prep Time: 30 minutes

Cook Time: 5 minutes

Ingredients:

- 1 large egg, separated
- Pinch cream of tartar
- Pinch salt
- 1 ounce cream cheese, softened
- 1 large egg
- 1 teaspoon butter
- 3 ounces sliced ham
- 1 slice cheddar cheese

Instructions:

1. For the bread, preheat the oven to 300°F and line a baking sheet with parchment.
2. Beat the egg whites with the cream of tartar and salt until soft peaks form.
3. Whisk the cream cheese and egg yolk until smooth and pale yellow.
4. Fold in the egg whites a little at a time until smooth and well combined.
5. Spoon the batter onto the baking sheet into two even circles.

6. Bake for 25 minutes until firm and lightly browned.
7. To complete the sandwich, fry the egg in butter until done to your preference.
8. Arrange the sliced ham on top of one bread circle.
9. Top with the fried egg and the sliced cheese then the second bread circle.
10. Serve immediately or cook in a greased skillet to melt the cheese first.

Nutrition Info: 530 calories, 40g fat, 36g protein, 5.5g carbs, 1g fiber, 4.5g net carbs

Lunch Recipes

Bacon-Wrapped Hot Dogs

Servings: 2

Prep Time: 10 minutes

Cook Time: 30 minutes

Ingredients:

- 4 all-beef hot dogs
- 2 slices cheddar cheese
- 4 slices uncooked bacon

Instructions:

1. Slice the hotdogs lengthwise, cutting halfway through the thickness.
2. Cut the cheese slices in half and stuff one half into each hot dog.
3. Wrap the hotdogs in bacon then place them on a foil-lined roasting pan.
4. Bake for 30 minutes or until the bacon is crisp.

Nutrition Info: 500 calories, 43g fat, 24g protein, 4g carbs, 0g fiber, 4g net carbs

Lunch Recipes

Fried Tuna Avocado Balls

Servings: 4

Prep Time: 10 minutes

Cook Time: 10 minutes

Ingredients:

- ¼ cup canned coconut milk
- 1 teaspoon onion powder
- 1 clove garlic, minced
- Salt and pepper

- 10 ounces canned tuna, drained
- 1 medium avocado, diced finely
- ½ cup almond flour
- ¼ cup olive oil

Instructions:

1. Whisk together the coconut milk, onion powder, garlic, salt and pepper in a bowl.
2. Flake the tuna into the bowl and stir in the avocado.
3. Divide the mixture into 10 to 12 balls and roll in the almond flour.
4. Heat the oil in a large skillet over medium-high heat.
5. Add the tuna avocado balls and fry until golden brown then drain on paper towels.

Nutrition Info: 455 calories, 38.5g fat, 23g protein, 8.5g carbs, 5g fiber, 3.5g net carbs

Lunch Recipes

Curried Chicken Soup

Servings: 4

Prep Time: 10 minutes

Cook Time: 20 minutes

Ingredients:

- 2 tablespoons olive oil, divided
- 4 boneless chicken thighs (about 12 ounces)
- 1 small yellow onion, chopped
- 2 teaspoons curry powder
- 2 teaspoons ground cumin
- Pinch cayenne
- 4 cups chopped cauliflower
- 4 cups chicken broth
- 1 cup water
- 2 cloves minced garlic
- ½ cup canned coconut milk
- 2 cups chopped kale
- Fresh chopped cilantro

Instructions:

1. Chop the chicken into bite-sized pieces then set aside.
2. Heat 1 tablespoon oil in a saucepan over medium heat.
3. Add the onions and cook for 4 minutes then stir in half of the spices.
4. Stir in the cauliflower and sauté for another 4 minutes.

5. Pour in the broth then add the water and garlic and bring to a boil.
6. Reduce heat and simmer for 10 minutes until the cauliflower is softened.
7. Remove from heat and stir in the coconut milk and kale.
8. Heat the remaining oil in a skillet and add the chicken – cook until browned.
9. Stir in the rest of the spices then cook until the chicken is done.
10. Stir the chicken into the soup and serve hot, garnished with fresh cilantro.

Nutrition Info: 390 calories, 22g fat, 34g protein, 14.5g carbs, 4.5g fiber, 10g net carbs

Lunch Recipes

Chopped Kale Salad with Bacon Dressing

Servings: 2

Prep Time: 15 minutes

Cook Time: None

Ingredients:

- 6 slices uncooked bacon
- 2 tablespoons apple cider vinegar
- 1 teaspoon Dijon mustard
- Liquid stevia, to taste
- Salt and pepper
- 4 cups fresh chopped kale
- ¼ cup thinly sliced red onion

Instructions:

1. Cook the bacon in a skillet until crisp then remove to paper towels and chop.
2. Reserve ¼ cup of the bacon grease in the skillet and warm over low heat.
3. Whisk in the apple cider vinegar, mustard, and stevia then season with salt and pepper.
4. Toss in the kale and cook for 1 minute then divide between two plates.
5. Top the salads with red onion and chopped bacon to serve.

Nutrition Info: 230 calories, 12g fat, 15g protein, 16g carbs, 2.5g fiber, 13.5g net carbs

Lunch Recipes

Kale Caesar Salad with Chicken

Servings: 2

Prep Time: 10 minutes

Cook Time: 10 minutes

Ingredients:

- 1 tablespoon olive oil
- 6 ounces boneless chicken thigh, chopped
- Salt and pepper
- 3 tablespoons mayonnaise
- 1 tablespoon lemon juice
- 1 anchovy, chopped
- 1 teaspoon Dijon mustard
- 1 clove garlic, minced
- 4 cups fresh chopped kale

Instructions:

1. Heat the oil in a skillet over medium-high heat.
2. Season the chicken with salt and pepper, then add to the skillet.
3. Cook until the chicken is no longer pink, then remove from heat.
4. Combine the mayonnaise, lemon juice, anchovies, mustard, and garlic in a blender.
5. Blend smooth, then season with salt and pepper.
6. Toss the kale with the dressing, then divide in half and top with chicken to serve.

Nutrition Info: 390 calories, 30g fat, 19g protein, 15g carbs, 2.5g fiber, 12.5g net carbs

Lunch Recipes

<u>Chicken Enchilada Soup</u>

Servings: 4

Prep Time: 15 minutes

Cook Time: 45 minutes

Ingredients:

- 2 tablespoons coconut oil
- 2 medium stalks celery, sliced
- 1 small yellow onion, chopped
- 1 small red pepper, chopped
- 2 cloves garlic, minced
- 1 cup diced tomatoes
- 2 teaspoons ground cumin
- 1 teaspoon chili powder
- ½ teaspoon dried oregano
- 4 cups chicken broth
- 1 cup canned coconut milk

- 8 ounces cooked chicken thighs, chopped
- 2 tablespoons fresh lime juice
- ¼ cup fresh chopped cilantro

Instructions:

1. Heat the oil in a saucepan over medium-high heat then add the celery, onion, peppers, and garlic – sauté for 4 to 5 minutes.
2. Stir in the garlic and cook for a minute until fragrant.
3. Add the tomatoes and spices then cook for 3 minutes, stirring often.
4. Add the broth and bring the soup to a boil, then reduce heat and simmer for about 20 minutes.
5. Stir in the coconut milk and simmer for another 20 minutes, then add the chicken.
6. Cook until the chicken is heated through, then stir in the lime juice and cilantro.

Nutrition Info: 380 calories, 27g fat, 24g protein, 12g carbs, 3.5g fiber, 8.5g net carbs

Lunch Recipes

Thai Coconut Shrimp Soup

Servings: 4

Prep Time: 10 minutes

Cook Time: 30 minutes

Ingredients:

- 1 tablespoon coconut oil
- 1 small yellow onion, diced
- 4 cups chicken broth
- 1 (14-ounce) can coconut milk
- 1 cup fresh chopped cilantro
- 1 jalapeno, seeded and chopped
- 1 tablespoon grated ginger
- 2 cloves garlic, minced
- 1 lime, zested and juiced
- 6 ounces uncooked shrimp, peeled and deveined
- 1 cup sliced mushrooms
- 1 small red onion, sliced thinly
- 1 tablespoon fish sauce

Instructions:

1. Heat the coconut oil in a saucepan over medium heat.
2. Add the yellow onions and sauté until translucent, about 6 to 7 minutes.
3. Stir in the chicken broth, coconut milk, cilantro, and jalapeno.
4. Add the ginger, garlic, and lime zest then bring to boil.
5. Reduce heat and simmer for 20 minutes - strain the mixture and discard the solids.
6. Return the remaining liquid to the saucepan and add the shrimp, mushrooms, and red onion.
7. Stir in the lime juice and fish sauce then simmer for 10 minutes. Serve hot.

Nutrition Info: 375 calories, 29.5g fat, 18g protein, 13g carbs, 3.5g fiber, 9.5g net carbs

Lunch Recipes

Mushroom and Asparagus Soup

Servings: 4

Prep Time: 10 minutes

Cook Time: 30 minutes

Ingredients:

- 1 tablespoon butter
- 1 small yellow onion, chopped
- 3 cloves garlic, minced
- 1 pound asparagus, trimmed and chopped
- 2 cups sliced mushrooms
- 4 cups vegetable broth
- 4 cups fresh baby spinach
- 1 teaspoon fresh chopped tarragon
- ½ cup heavy cream
- ¼ cup fresh lemon juice
- ¼ cup fresh chopped parsley
- Salt and pepper

Instructions:

1. Melt the butter in a stockpot and add the onion.
2. Sauté the onion until browned, then stir in the garlic and cook 1 minute more.
3. Stir in the asparagus and mushrooms, then sauté for 4 minutes.
4. Pour in the vegetable broth along with the spinach and tarragon.
5. Bring to a boil, then reduce heat and simmer for 30 minutes on medium-low heat.
6. Remove from heat, then stir in the cream, lemon juice, and parsley.
7. Cover and let rest for 20 minutes, then season with salt and pepper to taste.

Nutrition Info: 170 calories, 10.5g fat, 10g protein, 11g carbs, 4g fiber, 7g net carbs

Lunch Recipes

<u>Slow-Cooker Chicken Fajita Soup</u>

Servings: 4

Prep Time: 10 minutes

Cook Time: 6 hours

Ingredients:

- 12 ounces chicken thighs
- 1 cup diced tomatoes
- 2 cups chicken stock
- ½ cup enchilada sauce
- 2 ounces chopped green chiles
- 1 tablespoon minced garlic
- 1 medium yellow onion, chopped
- 1 small red pepper, chopped
- 1 jalapeno, seeded and minced
- 2 teaspoons chili powder
- ¾ teaspoon paprika
- ½ teaspoon ground cumin
- Salt and pepper
- 1 small avocado, sliced thinly
- ¼ cup chopped cilantro
- 1 lime, cut into wedges

Instructions:

1. Combine the chicken, tomatoes, chicken stock, enchilada sauce, chiles, and garlic in the slow cooker and stir well.
2. Add the onion, bell peppers, and jalapeno.
3. Stir in the seasonings then cover and cook on low for 5 to 6 hours.
4. Remove the chicken and chop or shred then stir it back into the soup.
5. Spoon into bowls and serve with sliced avocado, cilantro, and lime wedges.

Nutrition Info: 325 calories, 17g fat, 28g protein, 17g carbs, 7g fiber, 10g net carbs

Lunch Recipes

Avocado Egg Salad on Lettuce

Servings: 2

Prep Time: 10 minutes

Cook Time: None

Ingredients:

- 4 large hardboiled eggs, cooled and peeled
- 1 small avocado, pitted and chopped
- 1 medium stalk celery, diced
- ¼ cup diced red onion
- 2 tablespoons fresh lemon juice
- Salt and pepper
- 4 cups chopped romaine lettuce

Instructions:

1. Coarsely chop the eggs into a bowl.
2. Toss in the avocado, celery, red onion, and lemon juice.
3. Season with salt and pepper then serve over chopped lettuce.

Nutrition Info: 375 calories, 30g fat, 15.5g protein, 15g carbs, 8g fiber, 7g net carbs

Lunch Recipes

Bacon-Wrapped Chicken Rolls

Servings: 2

Prep Time: 5 minutes

Cook Time: 35 minutes

Ingredients:

- 6 boneless, skinless, chicken breast halves
- 6 slices uncooked bacon

Instructions:

1. Preheat the oven to 350°F.
2. Pound the chicken breast halves with a meat mallet to flatten.
3. Roll the chicken breast halves up then wrap each one with bacon.
4. Place the rolls on a foil-lined baking sheet.

5. Bake for 30 to 35 minutes until the chicken is done and the bacon crisp.

Nutrition Info: 350 calories, 16g fat, 46g protein, 0.5g carbs, 0g fiber, 0.5g net carbs

Lunch Recipes

<u>Spicy Shrimp and Sausage Soup</u>

Servings: 4

Prep Time: 15 minutes

Cook Time: 30 minutes

Ingredients:

- 1 tablespoon olive oil
- 3 small stalks celery, diced
- 1 small yellow onion, chopped
- 1 small red pepper, chopped
- 3 cloves garlic, minced
- 1 tablespoon tomato paste
- 2 teaspoons smoked paprika
- ½ teaspoon ground coriander
- Salt and pepper
- 8 ounces chorizo sausage, diced
- 1 cup diced tomatoes
- 4 cups chicken broth
- 12 ounces shrimp, peeled and deveined
- Fresh chopped cilantro

Instructions:

1. Heat the oil in a heavy stockpot over medium-high heat.
2. Add the celery, onion, and red pepper, and sauté for 6 to 8 minutes until tender.
3. Stir in the garlic, tomato paste, and seasonings, then cook for 1 minute.
4. Add the sausage and tomatoes and cook for 5 minutes.
5. Stir in the broth, then bring to a simmer and cook, uncovered, for 20 minutes.
6. Adjust seasoning to taste then add the shrimp.
7. Simmer until just cooked through, about 3 to 4 minutes.
8. Spoon into bowls and serve with fresh cilantro.

Nutrition Info: 465 calories, 28.5g fat, 39g protein, 11.5g carbs, 2g fiber, 9.5g net carbs

Lunch Recipes

<u>Slow-Cooker Beef Chili</u>

Servings: 4

Prep Time: 10 minutes

Cook Time: 6 hours

Ingredients:

- 1 tablespoon coconut oil
- 1 medium yellow onion, chopped
- 3 cloves garlic, minced
- 1 pound ground beef (80% lean)
- 1 small red pepper, chopped
- 1 small green pepper, chopped
- 1 cup diced tomatoes
- 1 cup low-carb tomato sauce
- 1 tablespoon chili powder
- 2 teaspoons dried oregano
- 1 ½ teaspoons dried basil
- Salt and pepper
- ¾ cup shredded cheddar cheese
- ½ cup diced red onion

Instructions:

1. Heat the oil in a skillet over medium-high heat.
2. Add the onions and sauté for 4 minutes, then stir in the garlic and cook 1 minute.
3. Stir in the beef and cook until it is browned, then drain some of the fat.
4. Spoon the mixture into a slow cooker and add the spices.
5. Cover and cook on low heat for 5 to 6 hours, then spoon into bowls.
6. Serve with shredded cheddar and diced red onion.

Nutrition Info: 395 calories, 19.5g fat, 42g protein, 12.5g carbs, 3.5g fiber, 9g net carbs

Dinner

Dinner Recipes

Grilled Pesto Salmon with Asparagus

Servings: 4

Prep Time: 5 minutes

Cook Time: 15 minutes

Ingredients:

- 4 (6-ounce) boneless salmon fillets
- Salt and pepper
- 1 bunch asparagus, ends trimmed
- 2 tablespoons olive oil
- ¼ cup basil pesto

Instructions:

1. Preheat a grill to high heat and oil the grates.
2. Season the salmon with salt and pepper, then spray with cooking spray.
3. Grill the salmon for 4 to 5 minutes on each side until cooked through.
4. Toss the asparagus with oil and grill until tender, about 10 minutes.
5. Spoon the pesto over the salmon and serve with the asparagus.

Nutrition Info: 300 calories, 17.5g fat, 34.5g protein, 2.5g carbs, 1.5g fiber, 1g net carbs

Dinner Recipes

Cheddar-Stuffed Burgers with Zucchini

Servings: 4

Prep Time: 10 minutes

Cook Time: 15 minutes

Ingredients:

- 1 pound ground beef (80% lean)
- 2 large eggs
- ¼ cup almond flour
- 1 cup shredded cheddar cheese
- Salt and pepper
- 2 tablespoons olive oil

- 1 large zucchini, halved and sliced

Instructions:

1. Combine the beef, egg, almond flour, cheese, salt, and pepper in a bowl.
2. Mix well, then shape into four even-sized patties.
3. Heat the oil in a large skillet over medium-high heat.
4. Add the burger patties and cook for 5 minutes until browned.
5. Flip the patties and add the zucchini to the skillet, tossing to coat with oil.
6. Season with salt and pepper and cook for 5 minutes, stirring the zucchini occasionally.
7. Serve the burgers with your favorite toppings and the zucchini on the side.

Nutrition Info: 470 calories, 29.5g fat, 47g protein, 4.5g carbs, 1.5g fiber, 3g net carbs

Dinner Recipes

Chicken Cordon Bleu with Cauliflower

Servings: 4

Prep Time: 10 minutes

Cook Time: 45 minutes

Ingredients:

- 4 boneless chicken breast halves (about 12 ounces)
- 4 slices deli ham
- 4 slices Swiss cheese
- 1 large egg, whisked well
- 2 ounces pork rinds
- ¼ cup almond flour
- ¼ cup grated parmesan cheese
- ½ teaspoon garlic powder
- Salt and pepper
- 2 cups cauliflower florets

Instructions:

1. Preheat the oven to 350°F and line a baking sheet with foil.
2. Sandwich the chicken breast halves between pieces of parchment and pound flat.
3. Lay the pieces out and top with sliced ham and cheese.
4. Roll the chicken up around the fillings then dip in the beaten egg.
5. Combine the pork rinds, almond flour, parmesan, garlic powder, salt and pepper in a food processor and pulse into fine crumbs.
6. Roll the chicken rolls in the pork rind mixture then place on the baking sheet.
7. Toss the cauliflower with melted butter then add to the baking sheet.

8. Bake for 45 minutes until the chicken is cooked through.

Nutrition Info: 420 calories, 23.5g fat, 45g protein, 7g carbs, 2.5g fiber, 4.5g net carbs

Dinner Recipes

<u>Sesame-Crusted Tuna with Green Beans</u>

Servings: 4

Prep Time: 15 minutes

Cook Time: 5 minutes

Ingredients:

- ¼ cup white sesame seeds
- ¼ cup black sesame seeds
- 4 (6-ounce) ahi tuna steaks
- Salt and pepper
- 1 tablespoon olive oil
- 1 tablespoon coconut oil
- 2 cups green beans

Instructions:

1. Combine the two types of sesame seeds in a shallow dish.
2. Season the tuna with salt and pepper.
3. Dredge the tuna in the sesame seed mixture.
4. Heat the olive oil in a skillet to high heat then add the tuna.
5. Cook for 1 to 2 minutes until seared then turn and sear on the other side.
6. Remove the tuna from the skillet and let the tuna rest while you reheat the skillet with the coconut oil.
7. Fry the green beans in the oil for 5 minutes then serve with sliced tuna.

Nutrition Info: 380 calories, 19g fat, 44.5g protein, 8g carbs, 3g fiber, 5g net carbs

Dinner Recipes

<u>Rosemary Roasted Pork with Cauliflower</u>

Servings: 4

Prep Time: 10 minutes

Cook Time: 20 minutes

Ingredients:

- 1 ½ pounds boneless pork tenderloin
- 1 tablespoon coconut oil
- 1 tablespoon fresh chopped rosemary
- Salt and pepper
- 1 tablespoon olive oil
- 2 cups cauliflower florets

Instructions:

1. Rub the pork with coconut oil, then season with rosemary, salt, and pepper.
2. Heat the olive oil in a large skillet over medium-high heat.
3. Add the pork and cook for 2 to 3 minutes on each side until browned.
4. Sprinkle the cauliflower in the skillet around the pork.
5. Reduce the heat to low, then cover the skillet and cook for 8 to 10 minutes until the pork is cooked through.
6. Slice the pork and serve with the cauliflower.

Nutrition Info: 300 calories, 15.5g fat, 37g protein, 3g carbs, 1.5g fiber, 1.5g net carbs

Dinner Recipes

Chicken Tikka with Cauliflower Rice

Servings: 6

Prep Time: 10 minutes

Cook Time: 6 hours

Ingredients:

- 2 pounds boneless chicken thighs, chopped
- 1 cup canned coconut milk
- 1 cup heavy cream
- 3 tablespoons tomato paste
- 2 tablespoons garam masala
- 1 tablespoon fresh grated ginger
- 1 tablespoon minced garlic
- 1 tablespoon smoked paprika
- 2 teaspoons onion powder
- 1 teaspoon guar gum
- 1 tablespoon butter
- 1 ½ cup riced cauliflower

Instructions:

1. Spread the chicken in a slow cooker, then stir in the remaining ingredients except for the cauliflower and butter.
2. Cover and cook on low heat for 6 hours until the chicken is done and the sauce thickened.
3. Melt the butter in a saucepan over medium-high heat.
4. Add the riced cauliflower and cook for 6 to 8 minutes until tender.
5. Serve the chicken tikka with the cauliflower rice.

Nutrition Info: 485 calories, 32g fat, 43g protein, 6.5g carbs, 1.5g fiber, 5g net carbs

Dinner Recipes

Grilled Salmon and Zucchini with Mango Sauce

Servings: 4

Prep Time: 5 minutes

Cook Time: 10 minutes

Ingredients:

- 4 (6-ounce) boneless salmon fillets
- 1 tablespoon olive oil
- Salt and pepper
- 1 large zucchini, sliced in coins
- 2 tablespoons fresh lemon juice
- ½ cup chopped mango
- ¼ cup fresh chopped cilantro
- 1 teaspoon lemon zest
- ½ cup canned coconut milk

Instructions:

1. Preheat a grill pan to high heat and spray liberally with cooking spray.
2. Brush the salmon with olive oil and season with salt and pepper.
3. Toss the zucchini with lemon juice and season with salt and pepper.
4. Place the salmon fillets and zucchini on the grill pan.
5. Cook for 5 minutes then turn everything and cook 5 minutes more.
6. Combine the remaining ingredients in a blender and blend into a sauce.
7. Serve the salmon fillets drizzled with the mango sauce and zucchini on the side.

Nutrition Info: 350 calories, 21.5g fat, 35g protein, 8g carbs, 2g fiber, 6g net carbs

Dinner Recipes

Slow-Cooker Pot Roast with Green Beans

Servings: 8

Prep Time: 10 minutes

Cook Time: 8 hours

Ingredients:

- 2 medium stalks celery, sliced
- 1 medium yellow onion, chopped
- 1 (3-pound) boneless beef chuck roast
- Salt and pepper
- ¼ cup beef broth
- 2 tablespoons Worcestershire sauce
- 4 cups green beans, trimmed
- 2 tablespoons cold butter, chopped

Instructions:

1. Combine the celery and onion in a slow cooker.
2. Place the roast on top and season liberally with salt and pepper.
3. Whisk together the beef broth and Worcestershire sauce then pour it in.
4. Cover and cook on low heat for 8 hours until the beef is very tender.
5. Remove the beef to a cutting board and cut into chunks.
6. Return the beef to the slow cooker and add the beans and chopped butter.
7. Cover and cook on high for 20 to 30 minutes until the beans are tender.

Nutrition Info: 375 calories, 13.5g fat, 53g protein, 6g carbs, 2g fiber, 4g net carbs

Dinner Recipes

Beef and Broccoli Stir-Fry

Servings: 4

Prep Time: 20 minutes

Cook Time: 15 minutes

Ingredients:

- ¼ cup soy sauce
- 1 tablespoon sesame oil
- 1 teaspoon garlic chili paste

- 1 pound beef sirloin
- 2 tablespoons almond flour
- 2 tablespoons coconut oil
- 2 cups chopped broccoli florets
- 1 tablespoon grated ginger
- 3 cloves garlic, minced

Instructions:

1. Whisk together the soy sauce, sesame oil, and chili paste in a small bowl.
2. Slice the beef and toss with almond flour, then place in a plastic freezer bag.
3. Pour in the sauce and toss to coat, then let rest for 20 minutes.
4. Heat the oil in a large skillet over medium-high heat.
5. Pour the beef and sauce into the skillet and cook until the beef is browned.
6. Push the beef to the sides of the skillet and add the broccoli, ginger, and garlic.
7. Sauté until the broccoli is tender-crisp, then toss it all together and serve hot.

Nutrition Info: 350 calories, 19g fat, 37.5g protein, 6.5g carbs, 2g fiber, 4.5g net carbs

Dinner Recipes

<u>Parmesan-Crusted Halibut with Asparagus</u>

Servings: 4

Prep Time: 10 minutes

Cook Time: 15 minutes

Ingredients:

- 1 pound asparagus, trimmed
- 2 tablespoons olive oil
- Salt and pepper
- ¼ cup butter, softened
- ¼ cup grated parmesan
- 2 tablespoons almond flour
- 1 teaspoon garlic powder
- 4 (6-ounce) boneless halibut fillets

Instructions:

1. Preheat the oven to 400°F and line a baking sheet with foil.
2. Toss the asparagus with olive oil and spread on the baking sheet.
3. Combine the butter, parmesan cheese, almond flour, garlic powder, salt, and pepper in a blender and blend until smooth.

4. Place the fillets on the baking sheet with the asparagus and spoon the parmesan mixture over the fish.
5. Bake for 10 to 12 minutes, then broil for 2 to 3 minutes until browned.

Nutrition Info: 415 calories, 26g fat, 42g protein, 6g carbs, 3g fiber, 3g net carbs

Dinner Recipes

Hearty Beef and Bacon Casserole

Servings: 8

Prep Time: 25 minutes

Cook Time: 30 minutes

Ingredients:

- 8 slices uncooked bacon
- 1 medium head cauliflower, chopped
- ¼ cup canned coconut milk
- Salt and pepper
- 2 pounds ground beef (80% lean)
- 8 ounces mushrooms, sliced
- 1 large yellow onion, chopped
- 2 cloves garlic, minced

Instructions:

1. Preheat the oven to 375°F.
2. Cook the bacon in a skillet until crisp, then drain on paper towels and chop.
3. Bring a pot of salted water to boil, then add the cauliflower.
4. Boil for 6 to 8 minutes until tender, then drain and add to a food processor with the coconut milk.
5. Blend the mixture until smooth, then season with salt and pepper.
6. Cook the beef in a skillet until browned, then drain the fat.
7. Stir in the mushrooms, onion, and garlic, then transfer to a baking dish.
8. Spread the cauliflower mixture over top and bake for 30 minutes.
9. Broil on high heat for 5 minutes, then sprinkle with bacon to serve.

Nutrition Info: 410 calories, 25.5g fat, 37g protein, 7.5g carbs, 3g fiber, 4.5g net carbs

Dinner Recipes

Sesame Wings with Cauliflower

Servings: 4

Prep Time: 5 minutes

Cook Time: 30 minutes

Ingredients:

- 2 ½ tablespoons soy sauce
- 2 tablespoons sesame oil
- 1 ½ teaspoons balsamic vinegar
- 1 teaspoon minced garlic
- 1 teaspoon grated ginger
- Salt
- 1 pound chicken wing, the wings itself
- 2 cups cauliflower florets

Instructions:

1. Combine the soy sauce, sesame oil, balsamic vinegar, garlic, ginger, and salt in a freezer bag, then add the chicken wings.
2. Toss to coat, then chill for 2 to 3 hours.
3. Preheat the oven to 400°F and line a baking sheet with foil.
4. Spread the wings on the baking sheet along with the cauliflower.
5. Bake for 35 minutes, then sprinkle with sesame seeds to serve.

Nutrition Info: 400 calories, 28.5g fat, 31.5g protein, 4g carbs, 1.5g fiber, 2.5g net carbs

Dinner Recipes

Fried Coconut Shrimp with Asparagus

Servings: 6

Prep Time: 15 minutes

Cook Time: 10 minutes

Ingredients:

- 1 ½ cups shredded unsweetened coconut
- 2 large eggs
- Salt and pepper
- 1 ½ pounds large shrimp, peeled and deveined

- ½ cup canned coconut milk
- 1 pound asparagus, cut into 2-inch pieces

Instructions:

1. Pour the coconut into a shallow dish.
2. Beat the eggs with some salt and pepper in a bowl.
3. Dip the shrimp first in the egg, then dredge with coconut.
4. Heat the coconut oil in a large skillet over medium-high heat.
5. Add the shrimp and fry for 1 to 2 minutes on each side until browned.
6. Remove the shrimp to paper towels and reheat the skillet.
7. Add the asparagus and season with salt and pepper – sauté until tender-crisp, then serve with the shrimp.

Nutrition Info: 535 calories, 38.5g fat, 29.5g protein, 18g carbs, 10g fiber, 8g net carbs

Dinner Recipes

Coconut Chicken Curry with Cauliflower Rice

Servings: 6

Prep Time: 15 minutes

Cook Time: 30 minutes

Ingredients:

- 1 tablespoon olive oil
- 1 medium yellow onion, chopped
- 1 ½ pounds boneless chicken thighs, chopped
- Salt and pepper
- 1 (14-ounce) can coconut milk
- 1 tablespoon curry powder
- 1 ¼ teaspoon ground turmeric
- 3 cups riced cauliflower

Instructions:

1. Heat the oil in a large skillet over medium heat.
2. Add the onions and cook until translucent, about 5 minutes.
3. Stir in the chicken and season with salt and pepper – cook for 6 to 8 minutes, stirring often, until browned on all sides.
4. Pour the coconut milk into the skillet, then stir in the curry powder and turmeric.
5. Simmer for 15 to 20 minutes until hot and bubbling.
6. Meanwhile, steam the cauliflower rice with a few tablespoons of water until tender.
7. Serve the curry over the cauliflower rice.

Nutrition Info: 430 calories, 29g fat, 33.5g protein, 9g carbs, 3.5g fiber, 5.5g net carbs

Dinner Recipes

<u>Spicy Chicken Enchilada Casserole</u>

Servings: 6

Prep Time: 15 minutes

Cook Time: 1 hour

Ingredients:

- 2 pounds boneless chicken thighs, chopped
- Salt and pepper
- 3 cups tomato salsa
- 1 ½ cups shredded cheddar cheese
- ¾ cup sour cream
- 1 cup diced avocado

Instructions:

1. Preheat the oven to 375°F and grease a casserole dish.
2. Season the chicken with salt and pepper then spread into the dish.
3. Spread the salsa over the chicken and sprinkle with cheese.
4. Cover with foil, then bake for 60 minutes until the chicken is done.
5. Serve with sour cream and chopped avocado.

Nutrition Info: 550 calories, 31.5g fat, 54g protein, 12g carbs, 4g fiber, 8g net carbs

Dinner Recipes

<u>White Cheddar Broccoli Chicken Casserole</u>

Servings: 6

Prep Time: 15 minutes

Cook Time: 30 minutes

Ingredients:

- 2 tablespoons olive oil
- 1 pound boneless chicken thighs, chopped
- 1 medium yellow onion, chopped
- 1 clove garlic, minced
- 1 ½ cups chicken broth
- 8 ounces cream cheese, softened

- ¼ cup sour cream
- 2 ½ cups broccoli florets
- ¾ cup shredded white cheddar cheese

Instructions:

1. Preheat the oven to 350°F and grease a casserole dish.
2. Heat the oil in a large skillet over medium-high heat.
3. Add the chicken and cook for 2 to 3 minutes on each side to brown.
4. Stir in the onion and garlic, and season with salt and pepper.
5. Sauté for 4 to 5 minutes until the chicken is cooked through.
6. Pour in the chicken broth, then add the cream cheese and sour cream.
7. Simmer until the cream cheese is melted, then stir in the broccoli.
8. Spread the mixture in the casserole dish and sprinkle with cheese.
9. Bake for 25 to 30 minutes until hot and bubbling.

Nutrition Info: 435 calories, 32g fat, 29.5g protein, 6g carbs, 1.5g fiber, 4.5g net carbs

Dinner Recipes

<u>Sausage Stuffed Bell Peppers</u>

Servings: 4

Prep Time: 15 minutes

Cook Time: 45 minutes

Ingredients:

- 1 medium head cauliflower, chopped
- 1 tablespoon olive oil
- 12 ounces ground Italian sausage
- 1 small yellow onion, chopped
- 1 teaspoon dried oregano
- Salt and pepper
- 4 medium bell peppers

Instructions:

1. Preheat the oven to 350°F.
2. Pulse the cauliflower in a food processor into rice-like grains.
3. Heat the oil in a skillet over medium heat then add the cauliflower – cook for 6 to 8 minutes until tender.
4. Spoon the cauliflower rice into a bowl, then reheat the skillet.
5. Add the sausage and cook until browned, then drain the fat.
6. Stir the sausage into the cauliflower, then add the onion, oregano, salt and pepper.

7. Slice the tops off the peppers, remove the seeds and pith, then spoon the sausage mixture into them.
8. Place the peppers upright in a baking dish, then cover the dish with foil.
9. Bake for 30 minutes, then uncover and bake 15 minutes more. Serve hot.

Nutrition Info: 355 calories, 23.5g fat, 19g protein, 16.5g carbs, 6g fiber, 10.5g net carbs

Dinner Recipes

Cheddar, Sausage, and Mushroom Casserole

Servings: 6

Prep Time: 15 minutes

Cook Time: 35 minutes

Ingredients:

- 1 pound ground Italian sausage
- 8 ounces mushrooms, diced
- 1 large yellow onion, chopped
- 1 cup shredded cheddar cheese
- 8 large eggs
- ½ cup heavy cream
- Salt and pepper

Instructions:

1. Preheat the oven to 375°F and grease a baking dish.
2. Heat the sausage in a large skillet over medium-high heat.
3. Cook the sausage until browned then stir in the mushrooms and onions.
4. Cook for 4 to 5 minutes then spread in the baking dish.
5. Sprinkle the dish with cheese then whisk together the remaining ingredients in a separate bowl.
6. Pour the mixture into the dish then bake for 35 minutes until bubbling.

Nutrition Info: 450 calories, 34g fat, 28g protein, 6g carbs, 1g fiber, 5g net carbs

Dinner Recipes

Cauliflower Crust Meat Lover's Pizza

Servings: 2

Prep Time: 20 minutes

Cook Time: 20 minutes

Ingredients:

- 1 tablespoon butter
- 2 cups riced cauliflower
- Salt and pepper
- 1 ½ cups shredded mozzarella cheese, divided into 1 cup and ½ cup
- 1 cup fresh grated parmesan
- 1 teaspoon garlic powder
- 1 large egg white
- 1 teaspoon dried Italian seasoning
- ¼ cup low-carb tomato sauce
- 2 ounces sliced pepperoni
- 1 ounce diced ham
- 2 slices bacon, cooked and crumbled

Instructions:

1. Preheat the oven to 400°F and line a baking sheet with parchment.
2. Heat the butter in a skillet over medium-high heat and add the cauliflower.
3. Season with salt and pepper, then cover and cook for 15 minutes, stirring occasionally, until very tender.
4. Spoon the cauliflower into a bowl and stir in ½ cup mozzarella along with the parmesan and garlic powder.
5. Stir in the egg white and Italian seasoning, then pour onto the baking sheet.
6. Shape the dough into a circle about ½-inch thick, then bake for 15 minutes.
7. Top with tomato sauce, along with the remaining mozzarella and the pepperoni, bacon, and ham.
8. Broil until the cheese is browned, then slice to serve.

Nutrition Info: 560 calories, 40.5g fat, 41g protein, 11g carbs, 3g fiber, 8g net carbs

Dinner Recipes

Slow Cooker Beef Bourguignon

Servings: 8

Prep Time: 15 minutes

Cook Time: 4 hours

Ingredients:

- 2 tablespoons olive oil
- 2 pounds boneless beef chuck roast, cut into chunks
- Salt and pepper

- ¼ cup almond flour
- ½ cup beef broth
- 2 cups red wine (dry)
- 2 tablespoons tomato paste
- 1 pound mushrooms, sliced
- 1 large yellow onion, cut into chunks

Instructions:

1. Heat the oil in a large skillet over medium-high heat.
2. Season the beef with salt and pepper, then toss with almond flour.
3. Add the beef to the skillet and cook until browned on all sides then transfer to a slow cooker.
4. Reheat the skillet over medium-high heat, then pour in the broth.
5. Scrape up the browned bits, then whisk in the wine and tomato paste.
6. Bring to a boil, then pour into the slow cooker.
7. Add the mushrooms and onion, then stir everything together.
8. Cover and cook on low heat for 4 hours until the meat is very tender. Serve hot.

Nutrition Info: 335 calories, 12.5g fat, 37.5g protein 6.5g carbs, 1.5g fiber, 5g net carbs

Dinner Recipes

<u>Pepper Grilled Ribeye with Asparagus</u>

Servings: 4

Prep Time: 5 minutes

Cook Time: 15 minutes

Ingredients:

- 1 pound asparagus, trimmed
- 2 tablespoons olive oil
- Salt and pepper
- 1 pound ribeye steak
- 1 tablespoon coconut oil

Instructions:

1. Preheat the oven to 400°F and line a small baking sheet with foil.
2. Toss the asparagus with olive oil and spread on the baking sheet.
3. Season with salt and pepper then place in the oven.
4. Rub the steak with the pepper and season with salt.
5. Melt the coconut oil in a cast-iron skillet and heat over high heat.
6. Add the steak and cook for 2 minutes then turn it.

7. Transfer the skillet to the oven and cook for 5 minutes or until the steak is done to the desired level.
8. Slice the steak and serve with the roasted asparagus.

Nutrition Info: 380 calories, 25g fat, 35g protein, 4.5g carbs, 2.5g fiber, 2g net carbs

Dinner Recipes

<u>Bacon-Wrapped Pork Tenderloin with Cauliflower</u>

Servings: 4

Prep Time: 10 minutes

Cook Time: 25 minutes

Ingredients:

- 1 ¼ pounds boneless pork tenderloin
- Salt and pepper
- 8 slices uncooked bacon
- 1 tablespoon olive oil
- 2 cups cauliflower florets

Instructions:

1. Preheat the oven to 425°F and season the pork with salt and pepper.
2. Wrap the pork in bacon and place on a foil-lined roasting pan.
3. Roast for 25 minutes until the internal temperature reaches 155°F.
4. Meanwhile, heat the oil in a skillet over medium heat.
5. Add the cauliflower and sauté until tender-crisp – about 8 to 10 minutes.
6. Turn on the broiler and place the pork under it to crisp the bacon.
7. Slice the pork to serve with the sautéed cauliflower.

Nutrition Info: 330 calories, 18.5g fat, 38g protein, 3g carbs, 1.5g fiber, 1.5g net carbs

Dinner Recipes

<u>Steak Kebabs with Peppers and Onions</u>

Servings: 4

Prep Time: 30 minutes

Cook Time: 10 minutes

Ingredients:

- 1 pound beef sirloin, cut into 1-inch cubes

- ¼ cup olive oil
- 2 tablespoons balsamic vinegar
- Salt and pepper
- 1 medium yellow onion, cut into chunks
- 1 medium red pepper, cut into chunks
- 1 medium green pepper, cut into chunks

Instructions:

1. Toss the steak cubes with the olive oil, balsamic vinegar, salt, and pepper.
2. Slide the cubes onto skewers with the peppers and onions.
3. Preheat a grill to high heat and oil the grates.
4. Grill the kebabs for 2 to 3 minutes on each side until done to your liking.

Nutrition Info: 350 calories, 20g fat, 35g protein, 6.5g carbs, 1.5g fiber, 5g net carbs

Dinner Recipes

Seared Lamb Chops with Asparagus

Servings: 4

Prep Time: 5 minutes

Cook Time: 15 minutes

Ingredients:

- 8 bone-in lamb chops
- Salt and pepper
- 1 tablespoon fresh chopped rosemary
- 1 tablespoon olive oil
- 1 tablespoon butter
- 16 spears asparagus, cut into 2-inch chunks

Instructions:

1. Season the lamb with salt and pepper then sprinkle with rosemary.
2. Heat the oil in a large skillet over medium-high heat.
3. Add the lamb chops and cook for 2 to 3 minutes on each side until seared.
4. Remove the lamb chops to rest and reheat the skillet with the butter.
5. Add the asparagus and turn to coat then cover the skillet.
6. Cook for 4 to 6 minutes until tender-crisp and serve with the lamb.

Nutrition Info: 380 calories, 18.5g fat, 48g protein, 4.5g carbs, 2.5g fiber, 2g net carbs

Dinner Recipes

Lemon Chicken Kebabs with Veggies

Servings: 4

Prep Time: 10 minutes

Cook Time: 15 minutes

Ingredients:

- 1 pound boneless chicken thighs, cut into cubes
- ¼ cup olive oil
- 2 tablespoons lemon juice
- 1 teaspoon minced garlic
- Salt and pepper
- 1 large yellow onion, cut into 2-inch chunks
- 1 large red pepper, cut into 2-inch chunks
- 1 large green pepper, cut into 2-inch chunks

Instructions:

1. Toss the chicken with the olive oil, lemon juice, garlic, salt, and pepper.
2. Slide the chicken onto skewers with the onion and peppers.
3. Preheat a grill to medium-high heat and oil the grates.
4. Grill the skewers for 2 to 3 minutes on each side until the chicken is done.

Nutrition Info: 360 calories, 21g fat, 34g protein, 8g carbs, 2g fiber, 6g net carbs

Dinner Recipes

Balsamic Salmon with Green Beans

Servings: 4

Prep Time: 15 minutes

Cook Time: 10 minutes

Ingredients:

- ½ cup balsamic vinegar
- ¼ cup chicken broth
- 1 tablespoon Dijon mustard
- 2 cloves garlic, minced
- 2 tablespoons coconut oil
- 4 (6-ounce) salmon fillets

- Salt and pepper
- 2 cups trimmed green beans

Instructions:

1. Combine the balsamic vinegar, chicken broth, mustard, and garlic in a small saucepan over medium-high heat.
2. Bring to a boil then reduce heat and simmer for 15 minutes to reduce by half.
3. Heat the coconut oil in a large skillet over medium-high heat.
4. Season the salmon with salt and pepper then add to the skillet.
5. Cook for 4 minutes until seared, then flip and add the green beans.
6. Pour the glaze into the skillet and simmer for 2 to 3 minutes until done.

Nutrition Info: 320 calories, 18g fat, 35g protein, 6g carbs, 2g fiber, 4g net carbs

Fat Bombs, Snacks And Desserts

Fat Bomb, Snack, and Dessert Recipes

Pumpkin Spiced Almonds

Servings: 4

Prep Time: 5 minutes

Cook Time: 25 minutes

Ingredients:

- 1 tablespoon olive oil
- 1 ¼ teaspoon pumpkin pie spice
- Pinch salt
- 1 cup whole almonds, raw

Instructions:

1. Preheat the oven to 300°F and line a baking sheet with parchment.
2. Whisk together the olive oil, pumpkin pie spice, and salt in a mixing bowl.
3. Toss in the almonds until evenly coated, then spread on the baking sheet.
4. Bake for 25 minutes then cool completely and store in an airtight container.

Nutrition Info: 170 calories, 15.5g fat, 5g protein, 5.5g carbs, 3g fiber, 2.5g net carbs

Fat Bomb, Snack, and Dessert Recipes

Coco-Macadamia Fat Bombs

Servings: 16

Prep Time: 5 minutes

Cook Time: None

Ingredients:

- 1 cup coconut oil
- 1 cup smooth almond butter
- ½ cup unsweetened cocoa powder
- ¼ cup coconut flour
- Liquid stevia extract, to taste
- 16 whole macadamia nuts, raw

Instructions:

1. Melt the coconut oil and cashew butter together in a small saucepan.
2. Whisk in the cocoa powder, coconut flour, and liquid stevia to taste.
3. Remove from heat and let cool until it hardens slightly.
4. Divide the mixture into 16 even pieces.
5. Roll each piece into a ball around a macadamia nut and chill until ready to eat.

Nutrition Info: 255 calories, 25.5g fat, 3.5g protein, 7g carbs, 3g fiber, 4g net carbs

Fat Bomb, Snack, and Dessert Recipes

Tzatziki Dip with Cauliflower

Servings: 6

Prep Time: 10 minutes

Cook Time: None

Ingredients:

- ½ (8-ounce) package cream cheese, softened
- 1 cup sour cream
- 1 tablespoon ranch seasoning
- 1 English cucumber, diced
- 2 tablespoons chopped chives
- 2 cups cauliflower florets

Instructions:

1. Beat the cream cheese with an electric mixer until creamy.
2. Add the sour cream and ranch seasoning, then beat until smooth.
3. Fold in the cucumbers and chives, then chill before serving with cauliflower florets for dipping.

Nutrition Info: 125 calories, 10.5g fat, 3g protein, 5.5g carbs, 1g fiber, 4.5g net carbs

Fat Bomb, Snack, and Dessert Recipes

Curry-Roasted Macadamia Nuts

Servings: 8

Prep Time: 5 minutes

Cook Time: 25 minutes

Ingredients:

- 1 ½ tablespoons olive oil
- 1 tablespoon curry powder
- ½ teaspoon salt
- 2 cups macadamia nuts, raw

Instructions:

1. Preheat the oven to 300°F and line a baking sheet with parchment.
2. Whisk together the olive oil, curry powder, and salt in a mixing bowl.
3. Toss in the macadamia nuts to coat, then spread on the baking sheet.
4. Bake for 25 minutes until toasted, then cool to room temperature.

Nutrition Info: 265 calories, 28g fat, 3g protein, 5g carbs, 3g fiber, 2g net carbs

Fat Bomb, Snack, and Dessert Recipes

Sesame Almond Fat Bombs

Servings: 16

Prep Time: 5 minutes

Cook Time: None

Ingredients:

- 1 cup coconut oil
- 1 cup smooth almond butter

- ½ cup unsweetened cocoa powder
- ¼ cup almond flour
- Liquid stevia extract, to taste
- ½ cup toasted sesame seeds

Instructions:

1. Combine the coconut oil and almond butter in a small saucepan.
2. Cook over low heat until melted, then whisk in the cocoa powder, almond flour, and liquid stevia.
3. Remove from heat and let cool until it hardens slightly.
4. Divide the mixture into 16 even pieces and roll into balls.
5. Roll the balls in the toasted sesame seeds and chill until ready to eat.

Nutrition Info: 260 calories, 26g fat, 4g protein, 6g carbs, 2g fiber, 4g net carbs

Fat Bomb, Snack, and Dessert Recipes

<u>Overnight Coconut Chia Pudding</u>

Servings: 6

Prep Time: 5 minutes

Cook Time: None

Ingredients:

- 2 ¼ cup canned coconut milk
- 1 teaspoon vanilla extract
- Pinch salt
- ½ cup chia seeds

Instructions:

1. Combine the coconut milk, vanilla, and salt in a bowl.
2. Stir well and sweeten with stevia to taste.
3. Whisk in the chia seeds and chill overnight.
4. Spoon into bowls and serve with chopped nuts or fruit.

Nutrition Info: 300 calories, 27.5g fat, 6g protein, 14.5g carbs, 10g fiber, 4.5g net carbs

Fat Bomb, Snack, and Dessert Recipes

<u>Chocolate Almond Butter Brownies</u>

Servings: 16

Prep Time: 15 minutes

Cook Time: 30 minutes

Ingredients:

- 1 cup almond flour
- ¾ cup unsweetened cocoa powder
- ½ cup shredded unsweetened coconut
- ½ teaspoon baking soda
- 1 cup coconut oil
- ½ cup canned coconut milk
- 2 large eggs
- 1 ½ teaspoons liquid stevia extract
- ¼ cup almond butter

Instructions:

1. Preheat the oven to 350°F and line a square pan with foil.
2. Whisk together the almond flour, cocoa powder, coconut, and baking soda in a mixing bowl.
3. In another bowl, beat together the coconut oil, coconut milk, eggs, and liquid stevia.
4. Stir the wet ingredients into the dry until just combined, then spread in the pan.
5. Melt the almond butter in the microwave until creamy.
6. Drizzle over the chocolate batter, then swirl gently with a knife.
7. Bake for 25 to 30 minutes until the center is set then cool completely, then cut into 16 equal pieces.

Nutrition Info: 200 calories, 21g fat, 3g protein, 4.5g carbs, 2.5g fiber, 2g net carbs

Fat Bomb, Snack, and Dessert Recipes

<u>Layered Almond Chocolate Fat Bombs</u>

Servings: 12

Prep Time: 10 minutes

Cook Time: None

Ingredients:

- ½ cup almond butter
- 6 tablespoons coconut oil, divided
- 1 teaspoon vanilla extract
- Liquid stevia extract, to taste
- 4 ounces 90% dark chocolate, chopped
- 1 ounce toasted almonds, finely chopped

Instructions:

1. Melt the almond butter and 2 tablespoons of coconut oil together in a bowl.
2. Stir in the vanilla extract and sweeten with stevia to taste.
3. Divide the mixture into 12 silicone baking molds and chill until set.
4. Melt the remaining coconut oil with the dark chocolate and stir until smooth.
5. Spoon into the silicone molds over the almond butter layer.
6. Sprinkle with chopped almonds and chill until solid.
7. Pop the fat bombs out of the molds and store in an airtight container in the fridge.

Nutrition Info: 160 calories, 16.5g fat, 2.5g protein, 4g carbs, 1.5g fiber, 2.5g net carbs

Fat Bomb, Snack, and Dessert Recipes

Bacon Cheeseburger Bites

Servings: 6

Prep Time: 5 minutes

Cook Time: 60 minutes

Ingredients:

- 12 ounces ground beef (80% lean)
- ½ cup diced yellow onion
- ½ teaspoon garlic powder
- Salt and pepper
- 12 slices uncooked bacon

Instructions:

1. Preheat the oven to 350°F and line a baking sheet with foil.
2. Stir the ground beef together with the onion, garlic powder, salt, and pepper.
3. Shape the mixture into twelve balls.
4. Wrap each ball in a slice of bacon and place on the baking sheet.
5. Bake for 50 to 60 minutes until the beef is cooked and bacon is crisp.

Nutrition Info: 215 calories, 11.5g fat, 24.5g protein, 1.5g carbs, 0.5g fiber, 1g net carbs

Fat Bomb, Snack, and Dessert Recipes

Layered Coco-Chia Fat Bombs

Servings: 12

Prep Time: 10 minutes

Cook Time: None

Ingredients:

- ½ cup coconut butter
- 6 tablespoons coconut oil, divided
- 2 tablespoons chia seeds
- ½ teaspoon coconut extract
- Liquid stevia extract, to taste
- 4 ounces 90% dark chocolate, chopped

Instructions:

1. Melt the coconut butter and 2 tablespoons of coconut oil together in a bowl.
2. Stir in the chia seeds and coconut extract, then sweeten with stevia to taste.
3. Divide the mixture into 12 silicone baking molds and chill until set.
4. Melt the remaining coconut oil with the dark chocolate and stir until smooth.
5. Spoon into the silicone molds over the solid layer and chill until solid.
6. Pop the fat bombs out of the molds and store in an airtight container in the fridge.

Nutrition Info: 215 calories, 21.5g fat, 2g protein, 6.5g carbs, 4.5g fiber, 2g net carbs

Fat Bomb, Snack, and Dessert Recipes

Cinnamon Quick Bread

Servings: 8

Prep Time: 10 minutes

Cook Time: 30 minutes

Ingredients:

- ½ cup coconut flour
- 1 ¼ teaspoon ground cinnamon

- 1 teaspoon baking soda
- ¼ teaspoon baking powder
- Pinch salt
- 6 tablespoons canned coconut milk
- 3 tablespoons melted coconut oil
- 2 tablespoons water
- 1 teaspoon apple cider vinegar
- 3 large eggs, whisked
- Liquid stevia extract

Instructions:

1. Preheat the oven to 350°F and grease a loaf pan.
2. Combine the coconut flour, cinnamon, baking soda, baking powder, and salt in a mixing bowl and stir well.
3. In another bowl, whisk together the coconut milk, oil, water, vinegar, and eggs.
4. Stir the wet ingredients into the dry, then sweeten to taste with stevia.
5. Spread the batter in the pan and cook for 25 to 30 minutes, then let cool.

Nutrition Info: 160 calories, 12g fat, 4.5g protein, 9g carbs, 5.5g fiber, 3.5g net carbs

Fat Bomb, Snack, and Dessert Recipes

<u>Lemon Meringue Cookies</u>

Servings: 8

Prep Time: 10 minutes

Cook Time: 60 minutes

Ingredients:

- 4 large egg whites
- Pinch salt
- Liquid stevia extract, to taste
- 1 teaspoon lemon extract

Instructions:

1. Preheat the oven to 225°F and line a baking sheet with parchment.
2. Beat the egg whites in a bowl until soft peaks form.
3. Add the salt and stevia, then beat until stiff peaks form.
4. Fold in the lemon extract, then spoon into a piping bag.
5. Pipe the mixture onto the baking sheet in small rounds.
6. Bake for 50 to 60 minutes until dry, then open the oven door and cool 20 minutes.

Nutrition Info: 10 calories, 0g fat, 2g protein, 0g carbs, 0g fiber, 0g net carbs

Fat Bomb, Snack, and Dessert Recipes

Almond Flour Cupcakes

Servings: 12

Prep Time: 10 minutes

Cook Time: 25 minutes

Ingredients:

- 2 ½ cups almond flour
- ¾ cup powdered erythritol
- 1 tablespoon baking powder
- ¼ teaspoon salt
- ¾ cup coconut oil, melted
- 3 large eggs
- 2 teaspoons vanilla extract

Instructions:

1. Preheat the oven to 350°F and line a muffin pan with paper liners.
2. In a bowl, whisk together the almond flour, erythritol, baking powder, and salt.
3. Whisk together the coconut oil, eggs, and vanilla in another bowl.
4. Combine the two mixtures and stir until just combined.
5. Spoon the batter into the prepared pan and bake for 22 to 25 minutes.
6. Let the cupcakes cool for 5 minutes in the pan, then turn out to cool completely.

Nutrition Info: 260 calories, 26g fat, 6g protein, 5g carbs, 2g fiber, 3g net carbs

Fat Bomb, Snack, and Dessert Recipes

Coconut Macaroons

Servings: 10

Prep Time: 10 minutes

Cook Time: 10 minutes

Ingredients:

- ½ cup unsweetened shredded coconut
- ¼ cup almond flour

- 2 tablespoons powdered erythritol
- 1 tablespoon coconut oil
- 1 teaspoon vanilla extract
- ½ teaspoon coconut extract
- 3 large egg whites

Instructions:

1. Preheat the oven to 400°F and line a baking sheet with parchment.
2. Combine the almond flour, coconut, and erythritol in a bowl.
3. In a separate bowl, melt the coconut oil, then whisk in the extracts.
4. Stir the two mixtures together until well combined.
5. Beat the egg whites in a bowl until stiff peaks form, then fold into the batter.
6. Spoon onto the baking sheet in even-sized mounds.
7. Bake for 7 to 9 minutes until the cookies are just browned on the edges.

Nutrition Info: 105 calories, 9g fat, 2.5g protein, 3g carbs, 2g fiber, 1g net carbs

Fat Bomb, Snack, and Dessert Recipes

<u>Vanilla Coconut Milk Ice Cream</u>

Servings: 6

Prep Time: 10 minutes

Cook Time: 30 minutes

Ingredients:

- 1 tablespoon coconut oil
- 2 cups canned coconut milk, divided
- Liquid stevia extract, to taste
- 1 teaspoon vanilla extract

Instructions:

1. Melt the coconut oil in a saucepan, then whisk in half of the coconut milk.
2. Bring to a boil, then reduce heat and simmer for 30 minutes.
3. Pour into a bowl and sweeten with stevia, then let cool to room temperature.
4. Stir in the vanilla extract, then pour the remaining coconut milk into a bowl.
5. Beat the coconut milk until stiff peaks form, then fold into the other mixture.
6. Spoon into a loaf pan and freeze until firm.

Nutrition Info: 205 calories, 21g fat, 2g protein, 4.5g carbs, 2g fiber, 2.5g net carbs

Fat Bomb, Snack, and Dessert Recipes

Crunchy Ginger Cookies

Servings: 16

Prep Time: 10 minutes

Cook Time: 15 minutes

Ingredients:

- 1 cup coconut butter
- 1 large egg
- 1 teaspoon vanilla extract
- ½ cup powdered erythritol
- ½ teaspoon ground ginger
- ½ teaspoon baking soda
- ¼ teaspoon ground nutmeg
- Pinch salt

Instructions:

1. Preheat the oven to 350°F and line a baking sheet with parchment.
2. Place the coconut butter in a food processor with the egg and vanilla.
3. Blend smooth then add the erythritol, ginger, baking soda, nutmeg, and salt.
4. Pulse until it forms a dough, then shape into 16 small balls.
5. Place the balls on the baking sheet and flatten slightly.
6. Bake for 12 to 15 minutes until the edges are browned then cool.

Nutrition Info: 190 calories, 18g fat, 2.5g protein, 7g carbs, 5g fiber, 2g net carbs

Fat Bomb, Snack, and Dessert Recipes

Vanilla Coconut Milk Flan

Servings: 4

Prep Time: 10 minutes

Cook Time: 1 hour

Ingredients:

- ½ cup heavy cream
- ½ cup whole milk
- ¼ cup powdered erythritol
- 1 tablespoon butter

- Pinch xanthan gum
- 2 large eggs
- ½ (14-ounce) can coconut milk
- 3 tablespoons shredded unsweetened coconut
- 1 teaspoon vanilla extract

Instructions:

1. Whisk together the heavy cream, milk, and erythritol in a saucepan then bring to a boil.
2. Cook on medium-low heat until reduced by half – about 1 hour.
3. Stir in the butter and xanthan gum, then remove from heat.
4. Preheat the oven to 325°F and grease 4 ramekins with butter or coconut oil.
5. Beat the eggs until frothy, then beat in the cream mixture along with the coconut milk, shredded coconut, and vanilla.
6. Adjust sweetness to taste, then divide among the four ramekins.
7. Bake for 50 to 60 minutes until the tops of the flans are lightly browned.
8. Cover with plastic and chill until ready to serve.

Nutrition Info: 260 calories, 25g fat, 6g protein, 5.5g carbs, 1.5g fiber, 4g net carbs

Fat Bomb, Snack, and Dessert Recipes

Peppermint Dark Chocolate Fudge

Servings: 16

Prep Time: 15 minutes

Cook Time: None

Ingredients:

- ½ cup coconut butter
- ⅓ cup coconut oil
- 4 ounces dark chocolate chips
- 1 teaspoon peppermint extract
- Liquid stevia extract, to taste

Instructions:

1. Combine the coconut butter, coconut oil, and dark chocolate in a double boiler over low heat.
2. Cook until the ingredients are melted, then stir until smooth.
3. Whisk in the peppermint extract and sweeten with stevia to taste.
4. Spread the mixture in a parchment-lined baking dish and chill until firm.
5. Remove the fudge from the dish and cut into squares to serve.

Nutrition Info: 165 calories, 15.5g fat, 1.5g protein, 8.5g carbs, 2.5g fiber, 6g net carbs

Fat Bomb, Snack, and Dessert Recipes

Layered Choco-Coconut Bars

Servings: 6

Prep Time: 20 minutes

Cook Time: None

Ingredients:

- 1 ½ cup shredded unsweetened coconut
- ½ cup canned coconut milk
- 1 teaspoon vanilla extract
- Liquid stevia extract
- 7 tablespoons coconut oil
- ¼ cup unsweetened cocoa powder

Instructions:

1. Combine the coconut, coconut milk, and vanilla in a bowl.
2. Stir well then sweeten with liquid stevia to taste.
3. Line a baking sheet with parchment and turn out the coconut mixture onto it – shape into a 4-by-6-inch rectangle.
4. Freeze for 2 hours until solid, then cut into six bars and set aside.
5. Melt the coconut oil in the microwave, then whisk in the cocoa powder and stevia to taste.
6. Cool the chocolate mixture slightly, then dip the bars in it until covered.
7. Place the bars on the baking sheet and chill to harden the chocolate.

Nutrition Info: 265 calories, 28g fat, 2g protein, 6g carbs, 3.5g fiber, 2.5g net carbs

Fat Bomb, Snack, and Dessert Recipes

Creamy Queso Dip

Servings: 8

Prep Time: 15 minutes

Cook Time: 5 minutes

Ingredients:

- 4 ounces chorizo, crumbled
- 1 clove garlic, minced

- ¼ cup heavy cream
- 6 ounces shredded white cheddar cheese
- 2 ounces shredded pepper jack cheese
- ¼ teaspoon xanthan gum
- Pinch salt
- 1 jalapeno, seeded and minced
- 1 small tomato, diced

Instructions:

1. Cook the chorizo in a skillet until evenly browned, then spoon into a bowl.
2. Reheat the skillet on medium-low heat and add the garlic – cook for 30 seconds.
3. Stir in the heavy cream, then add the cheese a little at a time, stirring often until it melts together.
4. Sprinkle with xanthan gum and salt, then stir well and cook until thickened.
5. Stir in the tomato and jalapeno, then serve with veggies for dipping.

Nutrition Info: 195 calories, 16g fat, 11g protein, 1.5g carbs, 0.5g fiber, 1g net carbs

Fat Bomb, Snack, and Dessert Recipes

Choco-Pistachio Fat Bombs

Servings: 16

Prep Time: 10 minutes

Cook Time: None

Ingredients:

- ½ cup coconut oil
- ½ cup coconut butter
- ¼ cup canned coconut milk
- ½ teaspoon vanilla extract
- Pinch salt
- ½ cup finely chopped pistachios
- 2 tablespoons unsweetened cocoa powder

Instructions:

1. Combine the coconut oil, coconut butter, and coconut milk in a large bowl.
2. Add the vanilla and salt, then beat on high speed until fluffy.
3. Transfer to the refrigerator and chill for an hour.
4. Scoop the mixture into 16 small portions and roll them into balls.
5. Combine the pistachios and cocoa powder in a bowl and roll the balls in it.
6. Chill until firm, then store in an airtight container.

Nutrition Info: 175 calories, 18g fat, 1.5g protein, 4.5g carbs, 3g fiber, 1.5g net carbs

Fat Bomb, Snack, and Dessert Recipes

Matcha Coconut Fat Bombs

Servings: 16

Prep Time: 10 minutes

Cook Time: None

Ingredients:

- ½ cup coconut oil
- ½ cup coconut butter
- ¼ cup canned coconut milk
- ½ teaspoon vanilla extract
- Pinch salt
- ½ cup shredded unsweetened coconut
- 2 teaspoons matcha powder

Instructions:

1. Combine the coconut oil, coconut butter, coconut milk, and a pinch of matcha powder in a large mixing bowl.
2. Add the vanilla and salt, then beat on high speed until fluffy.
3. Transfer to the refrigerator and chill for an hour.
4. Scoop the mixture into 16 small portions and roll them into balls.
5. Combine the coconut and matcha in a bowl and roll the balls in it.
6. Chill until firm, then store in an airtight container.

Nutrition Info: 170 calories, 17.5g fat, 1.5g protein, 4g carbs, 3g fiber, 1g net carbs

Fat Bomb, Snack, and Dessert Recipes

Coco-Almond Fat Bomb Bars

Servings: 12

Prep Time: 10 minutes

Cook Time: None

Ingredients:

- ½ cup cocoa butter
- ¼ cup unsweetened cocoa powder

- ¼ cup powdered erythritol
- 2 cups toasted almonds, chopped
- ½ cup heavy cream

Instructions:

1. Melt the cocoa butter in a small saucepan over low heat.
2. Whisk in the cocoa powder and sweeten with erythritol.
3. Stir in the chopped almonds and heavy cream until well combined.
4. Pour the mixture into silicone molds and let cool.
5. Transfer the molds to the fridge and chill until hardened.
6. Pop the fat bombs out of the molds and store in an airtight container.

Nutrition Info: 205 calories, 20.5g fat, 4.5g protein, 5g carbs, 3g fiber, 2g net carbs

Fat Bomb, Snack, and Dessert Recipes

Chocolate-Dipped Pecan Fat Bombs

Servings: 16

Prep Time: 10 minutes

Cook Time: None

Ingredients:

- 1 cup coconut butter
- 1 cup canned coconut milk
- 1 cup finely chopped pecans
- 1 teaspoon vanilla extract
- Liquid stevia extract, to taste
- ¼ cup chopped dark chocolate
- ½ teaspoon palm shortening

Instructions:

1. Combine the coconut butter and coconut milk in a small saucepan over low heat.
2. When melted, stir in the pecans and vanilla, then sweeten to taste.
3. Remove from heat and chill for 1 to 2 hours until firm.
4. Divide the mixture into 16 portions and roll them into small balls.
5. Melt the dark chocolate in the microwave with the palm shortening.
6. Dip the balls in the chocolate and place them on a plate.
7. Chill until the chocolate is hardened, then serve.

Nutrition Info: 245 calories, 24.5g fat, 3g protein, 9.5g carbs, 5.5g fiber, 4g net carbs

Fat Bomb, Snack, and Dessert Recipes

<u>Dark Chocolate Pistachio Fat Bombs</u>

Servings: 16

Prep Time: 10 minutes

Cook Time: None

Ingredients:

- 1 cup coconut butter
- 1 cup canned coconut milk
- 1 cup finely chopped pistachios
- 1 teaspoon vanilla extract
- Liquid stevia extract, to taste
- ¼ cup chopped dark chocolate
- ½ teaspoon palm shortening

Instructions:

1. Combine the coconut butter and coconut milk in a small saucepan over low heat.
2. When melted, stir in all but 1 tablespoon of the pistachios along with the vanilla then sweeten to taste.
3. Remove from heat and chill for 1 to 2 hours until firm.
4. Divide the mixture into 16 portions and roll them into small balls.
5. Melt the dark chocolate in the microwave with the palm shortening.
6. Dip the balls in the chocolate and place them on a plate.
7. Sprinkle with the remaining pistachios, then chill until the chocolate is hardened then serve.

Nutrition Info: 250 calories, 24g fat, 3g protein, 10g carbs, 6g fiber, 4g net carbs

Fat Bomb, Snack, and Dessert Recipes

<u>Chocolate-Dipped Coconut Fat Bombs</u>

Servings: 16

Prep Time: 10 minutes

Cook Time: None

Ingredients:

- 1 cup coconut butter
- 1 cup canned coconut milk

- ¾ cup unsweetened shredded coconut
- 2 teaspoons vanilla extract
- Liquid stevia extract, to taste
- ¼ cup chopped dark chocolate
- ½ teaspoon palm shortening

Instructions:

1. Combine the coconut butter and coconut milk in a small saucepan over low heat.
2. When melted, stir in the coconut and vanilla, then sweeten to taste.
3. Remove from heat and chill for 1 to 2 hours until firm.
4. Divide the mixture into 16 portions and roll them into small balls.
5. Melt the dark chocolate in the microwave with the palm shortening.
6. Dip the balls in the chocolate and place them on a plate.
7. Chill until the chocolate is hardened, then serve.

Nutrition Info: 300 calories, 28g fat, 3g protein, 11.5g carbs, 7g fiber, 4.5g net carbs

Fat Bomb, Snack, and Dessert Recipes

Chocolate Sunbutter Fat Bombs

Servings: 16

Prep Time: 5 minutes

Cook Time: None

Ingredients:

- 1 cup coconut oil
- 1 cup sunflower seed butter
- ½ cup unsweetened cocoa powder, divided
- ¼ cup coconut flour
- Liquid stevia extract, to taste

Instructions:

1. Melt the coconut oil and sunflower seed butter together in a small saucepan.
2. Whisk in ¼ cup of the cocoa powder along with the coconut flour, and liquid stevia to taste.
3. Remove from heat and let cool until it hardens slightly.
4. Divide the mixture into 16 even pieces and roll into balls then place on a plate.
5. Roll the fat bombs in the remaining cocoa powder to coat and chill.

Nutrition Info: 230 calories, 22g fat, 4g protein, 8g carbs, 2g fiber, 6g net carbs

Fat Bomb, Snack, and Dessert Recipes

Cinnamon Mug Cake

Servings: 1

Prep Time: 5 minutes

Cook Time: 1 minute

Ingredients:

- ⅓ cup almond flour
- 1 tablespoon powdered erythritol
- ½ teaspoon baking powder
- ¼ teaspoon ground cinnamon
- Pinch salt
- 1 large egg
- 1 tablespoon water
- 1 tablespoon coconut oil
- ½ teaspoon vanilla extract

Instructions:

1. Combine the almond flour, erythritol, baking powder, cinnamon, and salt.
2. In a separate bowl, whisk together the egg, water, coconut oil, and vanilla.
3. Stir the two mixtures together and pour into a greased coffee mug.
4. Cook in the microwave on high for 1 minute until done. Serve warm.

Nutrition Info: 395 calories, 36g fat, 13.5g protein, 8.5g carbs, 4g fiber, 4.5g net carbs

Fat Bomb, Snack, and Dessert Recipes

Raspberry Coconut Mousse

Servings: 6

Prep Time: 15 minutes

Cook Time: None

Ingredients:

- 1 ½ cup cashews, raw
- 3 tablespoons lemon juice
- 3 tablespoons water
- 1 ½ tablespoons coconut oil, melted
- 1 cup canned coconut milk (solids only)

- 1 teaspoon vanilla extract
- Liquid stevia extract, to taste
- ½ cup fresh raspberries, mashed slightly

Instructions:

1. Combine the cashews, lemon juice, water, and coconut oil in a blender and blend until smooth.
2. Beat the coconut milk with a hand mixer until stiff peaks form, then beat in the vanilla and stevia to taste.
3. Fold the whipped coconut milk into the cashew mixture then fold in the berries.
4. Spoon into jars and chill for at least 1 hour before serving.

Nutrition Info: 325 calories, 29g fat, 6.5g protein, 15g carbs, 2.5g fiber, 12.5g net carbs

Fat Bomb, Snack, and Dessert Recipes

<u>Chocolate Coconut Truffles</u>

Servings: 12

Prep Time: 15 minutes

Cook Time: None

Ingredients:

- 1 cup coconut butter
- 6 tablespoons unsweetened cocoa powder
- 2 tablespoons unsweetened shredded coconut
- 2 tablespoons instant coffee powder
- Liquid stevia extract, to taste
- 2 tablespoons coconut oil, melted

Instructions:

1. Melt the coconut butter in the microwave and stir until smooth.
2. Stir in the cocoa powder, coconut, coffee powder, and stevia.
3. Grease the cups of an ice cube tray with melted coconut oil.
4. Spoon the chocolate coconut mixture into the ice cube tray and pat down.
5. Freeze for 4 hours or until solid, then defrost for 15 minutes before serving.

Nutrition Info: 290 calories, 28g fat, 3.5g protein, 11g carbs, 8g fiber, 3g net carbs

Fat Bomb, Snack, and Dessert Recipes

<u>Cinnamon-Spiced Pumpkin Bars</u>

Servings: 6

Prep Time: 15 minutes

Cook Time: None

Ingredients:

- ½ cup coconut oil
- 4 ounces cream cheese, softened
- ¼ cup powdered erythritol
- 1 ½ teaspoons ground cinnamon
- ¼ cup pumpkin puree

Instructions:

1. Combine the coconut oil and cream cheese in a saucepan over medium-low heat.
2. Melt the ingredients, then stir well – transfer to a mixing bowl.
3. Beat in the erythritol and cinnamon, then spread in a dish lined with parchment.
4. Drizzle the pumpkin puree over the mixture and swirl with a knife.
5. Chill for 4 hours or until solid, then cut into bars to serve.

Nutrition Info: 225 calories, 25g fat, 1.5g protein, 2g carbs, 0.5g fiber, 1.5g net carbs

Fat Bomb, Snack, and Dessert Recipes

<u>Chocolate Avocado Pudding</u>

Servings: 4

Prep Time: 10 minutes

Cook Time: None

Ingredients:

- 2 medium avocados, pitted and chopped
- ½ cup heavy cream
- 2 tablespoons unsweetened cocoa powder
- 2 to 3 tablespoons powdered erythritol
- 1 tablespoon almond flour
- 1 teaspoon vanilla extract

Instructions:

1. Combine the ingredients in a food processor and pulse.
2. Blend on high speed until smooth, then spoon into cups.
3. Chill until thick and cold, then serve.

Nutrition Info: 275 calories, 26.5g fat, 3g protein, 11g carbs, 8g fiber, 3g net carbs

Fat Bomb, Snack, and Dessert Recipes

Classic Guacamole Dip

Servings: 4

Prep Time: 15 minutes

Cook Time: None

Ingredients:

- 2 medium avocado, pitted
- 1 small yellow onion, diced
- 1 small tomato, diced
- ¼ cup fresh chopped cilantro
- 1 tablespoon fresh lime juice
- 1 jalapeno, seeded and minced
- 1 clove garlic, minced
- Salt
- Sliced veggies to serve

Instructions:

1. Spoon the avocado flesh into a bowl and mash slightly.
2. Stir in the onion, tomato, cilantro, lime juice, garlic, and jalapeno.
3. Season with salt to taste and spoon into a bowl – serve with sliced veggies.

Nutrition Info: 220 calories, 20g fat, 2.5g protein, 12g carbs, 7.5g fiber, 4.5g net carbs

Fat Bomb, Snack, and Dessert Recipes

Cashew Macadamia Fat Bomb Bars

Servings: 16

Prep Time: 10 minutes

Cook Time: None

Ingredients:

- ½ cup almond butter
- ¼ cup unsweetened cocoa powder
- ¼ cup powdered erythritol
- 2 cups chopped macadamia nuts
- ½ cup heavy cream

Instructions:

1. Melt the almond butter in a small saucepan over low heat.
2. Whisk in the cocoa powder and sweeten with erythritol.
3. Stir in the chopped macadamia nuts and heavy cream until well combined.
4. Pour the mixture into silicone molds and let cool.
5. Transfer the molds to the fridge and chill until hardened.
6. Pop the fat bombs out of the molds and store in an airtight container.

Nutrition Info: 185 calories, 19.5g fat, 2.5g protein, 4.5g carbs, 2.5g fiber, 2g net carbs

With over 100 recipes contained herein, the whole idea here is to give you a boost in terms of the choice of food that you will get to enjoy beyond the 28-day meal plan provided. Designed to give the beginner an easier time while starting the keto diet, you will find that the meal plan gradually introduces the recipes, in an easy to follow format for you to prepare keto friendly, delicious foods that will serve you well on this ketogenic weight loss journey.

Once you have completed the meal plan, please feel free to mix and match the recipes here to create your very own meal plans! Always remember to keep the macronutrient numbers in mind and do not go overboard with the daily calorie intake. Eating too much can still pack on the pounds, whether you are on keto or not.

Conclusion:
Time To Take Action And Get Ketogenic

One of the main keys to any successful diet or lifestyle change has always been the recipes that fit in with the principles of the diet. I am sure there are many ways to achieve ketosis, and to attain that weight loss goal. However, you definitely do not want to get there by just having the same old dishes over and over again.

Variety is the name of the game here, which is crucial in ensuring the sustainability of the ketogenic diet. With the flavorful and delicious recipes found in this step by step keto cookbook, they will be useful additions for any keto dieter at any stage of their ketogenic journey. I have yet to see anyone complain about having too many easy yet delicious recipes!

For the beginners who have gotten this recipe cookbook, it would be quite useful for you to take the 28-day meal plan as a helpful guide, but you should definitely step out from that comfort zone sooner or later as you progress along your keto adventure! This is what the multiple recipes are for, so that you can pick and choose those which are most attractive to your palate.

For the more seasoned keto journeymen, do remember to make use of the recipe cards that are easily downloadable in the earlier sections. Just in case that slipped your mind, here is the link again.

Come Here To Get Your Recipe Cards
www.fcmediapublishing.com/recipecardsjkm2

Those cards are easy references and helpful buddies when you are in the kitchen, and even if you were to accidentally spill stuff or just damage them, you can easily print them out again! Maybe this time round, add on a layer of plastic laminate and the cards should be safe from spilt foods and liquids!

A Final Note

Phwoah! We have arrived at this juncture and I am so glad that you have chosen to take the steps needed on this ketogenic journey. This book and its contents, I hope, will be able to give you step by step actionable value, as always, for your progress toward nutritional ketosis.

More importantly, it is also my hope that the book has also given you the confidence booster and has built up your commitment to stay on the diet. Like I said in my other book, *Ketogenic Diet. The Step by Step Guide for Beginners: Optimal Path to Effective Weight Loss*, the benefits of ketosis await, and if health is wealth, you should be getting wealthy pretty soon!

There will be other books coming out on the ketogenic diet from me, so do look out for them. In the meantime, if you have enjoyed this book, please leave a review for me on Amazon and I would be most grateful!

Thank you, stay healthy and happy! Once again, thank you!

About the Author.

Jamie Moore has always been fascinated by food and what it can do for the human body since young, so much so that he ended up putting on so much weight that the doctors' advice at one point was for him to be wheel chair bound because any physical activity was deemed too strenuous for him. Yes, even walking! Things came to a head after one particularly bad hospital episode and that triggered the process to finally shed the unwanted pounds.

It wasn't an easy road. Despite going on varying diets, weight loss regimes and spending on the latest exercise gear, the results just weren't manifesting itself. It wasn't until Jamie chanced upon the ketogenic diet that things got turned around for the better. Enthralled with what he had found and his own positive experiences with the diet for weight loss, Jamie took up distance learning courses to get accreditation on dieting and nutrition in order to further understand more about the ketogenic diet.

That was many years ago. These days, Jamie does forty laps in the pool with regular gym sessions thrown in for good measure. He does not term himself as a health geek, but most of his friends beg to differ! They come to him for anything on diet, nutrition and exercise. That was also part of the reason why Jamie took to penning down what he knew into books which he hopes would be of help to people.

Appendix A: The Grocery Lists

Standard 28-Day Meal Plan: Shopping List Week 1

Meat, Eggs, and Seafood

- Bacon, thick-cut – 24 slices
- Beef, ground (80% lean) – 30 ounces
- Chicken thighs, boneless – 2 pounds
- Eggs – 17 large
- Ham, deli, sliced – 3 ounces
- Ham, fat-free – 6 ounces
- Salmon, boneless – 4 (6-ounce) fillets

Fruits and Vegetables

- Asparagus – 1 bunch
- Avocado – 3 small, 3 medium
- Beets – 1 small
- Bell pepper, red – 1 small
- Cauliflower – 2 cups
- Chives – 1 bunch
- Cucumber, English – 1 ½ medium
- Garlic – 1 head
- Kale – 1 cup
- Lemon – 1
- Lettuce – 5 cups
- Mushrooms – 1 cup
- Onion, red – 1 small
- Onion, yellow – 1 small, 1 medium
- Spinach – 2 cups
- Tomatoes – ½ cup
- Zucchini – 1 small, 1 large

Refrigerated and Frozen Goods

- Almond milk, unsweetened – 1 ¾ cups
- Blueberries, frozen – ¼ cup
- Cheddar cheese, shredded – 1 ¾ cups
- Coconut milk, unsweetened – 1 cup
- Cream cheese – 9 ounces
- Heavy cream – ¼ cup
- Mayonnaise – 3 tablespoons

- Parmesan cheese, grated – 1 cup
- Provolone cheese, shredded – ¼ cup
- Sour cream – 1 cup
- Yogurt, full-fat – ¾ cup

Pantry Staples and Dry Goods

- Almonds, whole – 1 cup
- Almond butter – 1 cup plus 1 tablespoon
- Almond flour – ½ cup
- Apple cider vinegar
- Basil pesto – ¼ cup
- Black pepper
- Broth, beef – 3 cups
- Chia seeds – 1 teaspoon
- Chili powder
- Cocoa powder, unsweetened
- Coconut flour – ¼ cup
- Coconut oil
- Cream of tartar
- Dijon mustard
- Ground cinnamon
- Ground cumin
- Olive oil
- Liquid stevia extract
- Macadamia nuts – 16 whole
- Paprika
- Powdered erythritol
- Protein powder, egg white, vanilla – ¼ cup
- Pumpkin pie spice
- Ranch seasoning
- Salt
- Tomato paste – 2 tablespoons

Standard 28-Day Meal Plan: Shopping List Week 2

Meat, Eggs, and Seafood

- Bacon, thick-cut – 19 slices
- Chicken thighs, boneless – 2 pounds
- Eggs – 26 large
- Ham, deli, diced – ¼ cup
- Ham, fat-free – 2 pounds plus 1 ounce
- Pork tenderloin, boneless – 1 ½ pounds
- Salmon, boneless – 8 ounces
- Tuna, ahi – 4 (6-ounce) steaks

Fruits and Vegetables

- Avocado – 2 small, 2 medium
- Bell pepper, green – 1 small
- Cauliflower – 3 cups
- Celery – 1 small stalk
- Garlic – 1 head
- Ginger – 1 piece
- Green beans – 2 cups
- Lemon – 1
- Lettuce – 4 ¼ cups
- Onion, red – 1 small
- Onion, yellow – 1 small
- Parsley – 1 bunch
- Rosemary – 1 bunch
- Spring greens – 4 ounces
- Tomato – 1 small

Refrigerated and Frozen Goods

- Almond milk, unsweetened – ¾ cup
- Butter – 1 tablespoon
- Cream cheese – 1 ounce
- Heavy cream – 1 cup plus 1 tablespoon
- Mayonnaise – 3 tablespoons
- Parmesan, shaved – ¼ cup

Pantry Staples and Dry Goods

- Almond butter – 1 ¾ cups
- Almond flour – 2 ½ cups
- Baking powder
- Black pepper
- Broth, chicken – 5 cups
- Chia seeds – ½ cup
- Chicken bouillon – 4 cubes
- Chili garlic paste
- Cocoa powder, unsweetened
- Coconut flour – 2 tablespoons
- Coconut milk, canned – 3 ¼ cups
- Coconut oil
- Cream of tartar
- Dijon mustard
- Egg white protein powder – 2 scoops (40g)
- Garam masala
- Ground cinnamon
- Ground nutmeg
- Guar gum
- Olive oil
- Onion powder
- Liquid stevia extract
- Pine nuts, roasted – ⅓ cup
- Powdered erythritol
- Red wine vinegar
- Salt
- Sesame seeds, black – ¼ cup
- Sesame seeds, toasted – ½ cup
- Sesame seeds, white – ¼ cup
- Smoked paprika
- Tomato paste – 3 tablespoons
- Vanilla extract

Standard 28-Day Meal Plan: Shopping List Week 3

Meat, Eggs, and Seafood

- Bacon, thick-cut – 30 slices
- Beef, boneless chuck roast – 3 pounds
- Beef, ground (80% lean) – 12 ounces
- Beef, sirloin – 1 pound
- Chicken breast, cooked – 1 cup
- Chicken tenders, boneless – 2 pounds
- Chicken thighs, boneless – 8 ounces
- Eggs – 18 large
- Ham, deli, diced – 2 cups
- Ham, fat-free – 12 ounces
- Salmon, boneless – 4 (6-ounce) fillets

Fruits and Vegetables

- Avocado – 1 small, 8 medium
- Broccoli – 2 cups
- Cauliflower – 2 cups
- Celery – 1 small, 2 medium stalks
- Cilantro – 1 bunch
- Garlic – 1 head
- Ginger – 1 piece
- Green beans – 4 cups
- Kale – 1 cup
- Lemon – 2
- Lime – 1
- Mango – 1 small
- Onion, yellow – 2 small, 1 medium
- Spinach – 8 ounces plus 5 cups
- Spring greens – 4 cups
- Zucchini – 1 large

Refrigerated and Frozen Goods

- Almond milk, unsweetened – ¾ cup
- Butter – 2 tablespoons
- Cashew milk, unsweetened – 1 cup
- Cream cheese – 1 ounce
- Heavy cream – ¼ cup
- Pepper jack cheese, shredded – 1 cup
- Swiss cheese – 1 slice

Pantry Staples and Dry Goods

- Almonds, sliced – 1 ounce plus 5 tablespoons
- Almond butter – ¾ cup
- Almond flour – 1 ⅓ cups
- Baking soda
- Balsamic vinegar
- Black pepper
- Broth, beef – ¼ cup
- Broth, vegetable – 3 cups
- Cocoa powder, unsweetened
- Coconut, shredded unsweetened – ¾ cup
- Coconut milk, canned – 1 ½ cups
- Coconut oil
- Cream of tartar
- Dark chocolate (90% cacao) – 4 ounces
- Dijon mustard
- Garlic chili paste
- Garlic powder
- Olive oil
- Liquid stevia extract
- Matcha powder – 1 teaspoon
- Powdered erythritol
- Pumpkin pie spice
- Pumpkin puree – ½ cup
- Rice wine vinegar
- Salt
- Sesame oil
- Sesame seeds – 1 tablespoon
- Soy sauce
- Vanilla extract
- Worcestershire sauce

Standard 28-Day Meal Plan: Shopping List Week 4

Meat, Eggs, and Seafood

- Bacon, thick-cut – 20 slices
- Beef, ground (80% lean) – 2 pounds
- Beef, sirloin – 8 ounces
- Chicken wing pieces – 1 pound
- Eggs – 30 large
- Halibut, boneless – 4 (6-ounce) fillets
- Ham, deli, diced – 1 cup
- Ham, deli, sliced – 1 ounce
- Ham, fat-free – 30 ounces
- Pancetta, diced – 2 ounces
- Salami – 1 ounce
- Turkey, sliced – 1 ounce
- Tuna, in oil – 2 (6-ounce) cans

Fruits and Vegetables

- Asparagus – 1 pound
- Avocado – 1 small, 5 medium
- Bell pepper, green – 1 small
- Bell pepper, red – 1 small
- Cauliflower – 2 medium heads
- Cucumber – ½ cup
- Garlic – 1 head
- Ginger – 1 piece
- Kale – 1 cup
- Leeks – 2 medium
- Lemon – 1
- Lettuce – 8 cups
- Mushrooms – 8 ounces
- Onion, green – 1 bunch
- Onion, yellow – 1 small, 1 large
- Tomato – 1 medium
- Tomatoes, cherry – 1 cup

Refrigerated and Frozen Goods

- Almond milk, unsweetened – ½ cup
- Broccoli, frozen – ¼ cup
- Butter – 5 tablespoons
- Cheddar cheese, shredded – ½ cup

- Cheddar cheese, sliced – 2 slices
- Cream cheese – 1 ounce
- Heavy cream – ½ cup plus 1 tablespoon
- Mayonnaise – ¼ cup
- Mozzarella cheese, shredded – 1 cup
- Parmesan, grated – 6 tablespoons

Pantry Staples and Dry Goods

- Almond flour – 2 tablespoons
- Apple cider vinegar
- Baking powder
- Baking soda
- Balsamic vinegar
- Black pepper
- Broth, chicken – 4 cups
- Chia seeds – 2 tablespoons
- Coconut, unsweetened, shredded – ¼ cup
- Coconut butter – ½ cup
- Coconut extract
- Coconut flour – 1 ¼ cups
- Coconut milk, canned – 1 cup
- Coconut oil
- Cream of tartar
- Dark chocolate (90% cacao) – 4 ounces
- Dijon mustard
- Garlic powder
- Ground cardamom
- Ground cinnamon
- Ground cloves
- Ground ginger
- Olive oil
- Liquid stevia extract
- Pickle relish
- Powdered erythritol
- Salt
- Sesame oil
- Soy sauce
- Vanilla extract

Appendix B: Conversion Charts

Weight Conversions		
Metric	**Cups**	**Ounces**
15g	1 tablespoon	½ ounce
30g	⅛ cup	1 ounce
60g	¼ cup	2 ounces
115g	½ cup	4 ounces
170g	¾ cup	6 ounces
225g	1 cup	8 ounces
450g	2 cups	16 ounces

Volume Conversions		
Metric	**Cups**	**Ounces**
15 ml	1 tablespoon	½ fluid ounce
30 ml	2 tablespoons	1 fluid ounce
60 ml	¼ cup	2 fluid ounces
125 ml	½ cup	4 fluid ounces
180 ml	¾ cup	6 fluid ounces
250 ml	1 cup	8 fluid ounces
500 ml	2 cups	16 fluid ounces
1,000 ml	4 cups	1 quart

Appendix C: Recipe Index

<u>A</u>

Almond Butter Muffins

Almond Butter Protein Smoothie

Almond Flour Cupcakes

Avocado Egg Salad on Lettuce

Avocado Spinach Salad with Almonds

<u>B</u>

Bacon Cheeseburger Bites

Bacon Cheeseburger Soup

Bacon Swiss Waffles

Bacon, Lettuce, Tomato, Avocado Sandwich

Bacon, Mushroom, and Swiss Omelet

Bacon-Wrapped Chicken Rolls

Bacon-Wrapped Hot Dogs

Bacon-Wrapped Pork Tenderloin with Cauliflower

Baked Chicken Nuggets

Balsamic Salmon with Green Beans

Beef and Broccoli Stir-Fry

Beef and Pepper Kebabs

Beets and Blueberry Smoothie

Broccoli Kale Egg Scramble

<u>C</u>

Cashew Macadamia Fat Bomb Bars

Cauliflower Crust Meat Lover's Pizza

Cauliflower Leek Soup with Pancetta

Cheddar, Sausage, and Mushroom Casserole

Cheddar-Stuffed Burgers with Zucchini

Cheesy Buffalo Chicken Sandwich

Chicken Cordon Bleu with Cauliflower

Chicken Enchilada Soup

Chicken Tikka with Cauliflower Rice

Chocolate Almond Butter Brownies

Chocolate Avocado Pudding

Chocolate Coconut Truffles

Chocolate Protein Pancakes

Chocolate Sunbutter Fat Bombs

Chocolate-Dipped Coconut Fat Bombs

Chocolate-Dipped Pecan Fat Bombs

Choco-Pistachio Fat Bombs

Chopped Kale Salad with Bacon Dressing

Cinnamon Almond Porridge

Cinnamon Mug Cake

Cinnamon Protein Pancakes

Cinnamon Quick Bread

Cinnamon Roll Waffles

Cinnamon-Spiced Pumpkin Bars

Classic Guacamole Dip

Classic Western Omelet

Coco-Almond Fat Bomb Bars

Coco-Cashew Macadamia Muffins

Coco-Macadamia Fat Bombs

Coconut Chicken Curry with Cauliflower Rice

Coconut Chicken Tenders

Coconut Macaroons

Creamy Chocolate Protein Smoothie

Creamy Queso Dip

Crispy Chai Waffles

Crunchy Ginger Cookies

Cucumber Avocado Salad with Bacon

Curried Chicken Soup

Curry-Roasted Macadamia Nuts

Coconut Chia Pudding

D

Dark Chocolate Pistachio Fat Bombs

Detoxifying Green Smoothie

E

Easy Chopped Salad

Egg Drop Soup

Egg Salad Over Lettuce

F

Fried Coconut Shrimp with Asparagus

Fried Salmon Cakes

Fried Tuna Avocado Balls

G

Grilled Pesto Salmon with Asparagus

Grilled Salmon and Zucchini with Mango Sauce

H

Ham and Provolone Sandwich

Ham, Cheddar, and Chive Omelet

Ham, Egg, and Cheese Sandwich

Hearty Beef and Bacon Casserole

K

Kale Avocado Smoothie

Kale Caesar Salad with Chicken

L

Layered Almond Chocolate Fat Bombs

Layered Choco-Coconut Bars

Layered Coco-Chia Fat Bombs

Lemon Chicken Kebabs with Veggies

Lemon Flaxseed Muffins

Lemon Meringue Cookies

M

Maple Cranberry Muffins

Matcha Coconut Fat Bombs

Meaty Breakfast Omelet

Mushroom and Asparagus Soup

N

Nutty Pumpkin Smoothie

P

Parmesan-Crusted Halibut with Asparagus

Pepper Grilled Ribeye with Asparagus

Peppermint Dark Chocolate Fudge

Pumpkin Spice Waffles

Pumpkin Spiced Almonds

R

Raspberry Coconut Mousse

Rosemary Roasted Pork with Cauliflower

S

Sausage Stuffed Bell Peppers

Seared Lamb Chops with Asparagus

Sesame Almond Fat Bombs

Sesame Chicken Avocado Salad

Sesame Wings with Cauliflower

Sesame-Crusted Tuna with Green Beans

Sheet Pan Eggs with Ham and Pepper Jack

Sheet Pan Eggs with Veggies and Parmesan

Simple Tuna Salad on Lettuce

Slow Cooker Beef Bourguignon

Slow-Cooker Beef Chili

Slow-Cooker Chicken Fajita Soup

Slow-Cooker Pot Roast with Green Beans

Spicy Chicken Enchilada Casserole

Spicy Shrimp and Sausage Soup

Spinach Cauliflower Soup

Spinach Parmesan Egg Scramble

Spring Salad with Shaved Parmesan

Steak Kebabs with Peppers and Onions

Strawberry Rhubarb Pie Smoothie

T

Taco Salad with Creamy Dressing

Thai Coconut Shrimp Soup

Three Cheese Egg Muffins

Three Meat and Cheese Sandwich

Tomato Mozzarella Egg Muffins

Tzatziki Dip with Cauliflower

V

Vanilla Chai Smoothie

Vanilla Coconut Milk Flan

Vanilla Coconut Milk Ice Cream

W

White Cheddar Broccoli Chicken Casserole

Made in United States
Troutdale, OR
08/09/2023